1987

Building a Better Hospital Board

John A. Witt

Building a Better Hospital Board

MANAGEMENT SERIES
American College of Healthcare Executives

Library of Congress Cataloging-in-Publication Data

Witt, John A.
    Building a better hospital board.

    Includes index.
    1. Hospitals—Trustees. 2. Hospitals—Administration. I. Title.
[DNLM: 1. Governing Board—organization & administration. 2.
Hospital Administration. WX 150 W827b]
RA971.W58 1987   362.1'1'068   87-21226
ISBN 0-910701-29-6

Health Administration Press
A Division of the Foundation of the
    American College of Healthcare Executives
1021 East Huron Street
Ann Arbor, Michigan 48104-9990
(313) 764-1380

For my parents,
whose love and encouragement, when they were with me,
made seeking and growth a way of life,

And Merton E. Knisely,
a former CEO of St. Luke's Hospital in Wisconsin, whose
visioneering in health care was a model,

And my wife, Carol,
who is also my best friend.

With appreciation and love.

Contents

7.

8.

9.

10.

11.

12.

Acknowledgments

How do I recognize and affirm the many people over the years who have contributed to this book? Some have done it by encouraging, cajoling, and pushing me in the first place. Others provided problems for solutions or ideas for stimulation and dialogue for formulating concepts. Still others gave me the opportunity to work with and for them.

Thank you, officers of Witt Associates, for allowing me the time to complete this task.

Thank you to Karen Kelly, for the many hours of effort to clarify, crystallize, and finalize copy that never seemed to stop changing.

Thank you to Edward Weimer and Edward Miller of the American Hospital Association, without whom I never could have started the research.

Thank you to Richard and Everett Johnson, for listening as the concepts evolved for this book.

Thank you to Joe Ryan, a former A. T. Kearney consultant, whose willingness to teach consulting as a vital, ethical service caused me to make it a career.

Finally, to the thousands of hospital board members in seminars, workshops, and consulting assignments who became involved in my education as well as their own, I say thank you.

JOHN A. WITT
August 1987

Introduction

Why was it this call and not one of the hundreds of others over the years? I don't know. When I took a call from a health care organization's board chairperson in June 1985, asking me to help him improve his board, what had been for years a simmering pot suddenly came to a boil.

As I spoke with that gentleman about his board's problems, I began to think about creating a means of conveying more widely what my 25 years as a consultant in the health care field have taught me about boards and their need for development.

I really believe it is possible to make a good board better. I am confident from my years as a speaker at board seminars and retreats that most boards *want* to become better. And I know that board chairpersons and their top management are eager to promote this growth. Therefore, I have written *Building a Better Hospital Board* to encourage people who are on hospital boards or working with hospital boards to think about how they could make their boards stronger and more effective.

This book is written for decision-making boards. Some groups function in an advisory capacity only; these groups are also called boards. One system of religious hospitals acknowledged, that its boards are not autonomous but for example, it considers them very valuable for quality assurance. Groups like that will need another book. This book is not for ceremonial boards but for working boards.

No book on this subject could specifically describe every board. As some read about other's weaknesses, they'll tend to feel this book is not for them because they're further along in their growth process. Others who really need help may rationalize that they are so unique, no one could have answers for their one-of-a-kind situations. I would just ask readers to digest the entire book and then reflect on *how*—not *whether*—their own boards can be strengthened. Because boards are groups of people, constantly changing, with greater or lesser experience, development needs will vary. But every board has the capacity to be better.

I've tried to keep in mind one key to developing a better health care organization board—that most board people are truly *volunteers*. They are giving their time freely; to suggest improvements may make some of the volunteers feel they are being unfairly criticized. I see my efforts less as criticism than as advice. My experience with hospital boards has impressed on me that many boards are ineffectual, although I'm convinced the situation can be improved.

The underlying principles in this book are derived from the need for voluntary boards to know themselves. My work with hospitals, professional associations, and the evolving, restructured health care corporations has convinced me that to be maximally effective, voluntary boards must see themselves as organisms that have lives of their own and unique patterns to their lives.

This understanding is needed even more by the new organizational forms that have been superimposed on the health care industry, compounding the problem of training board members by simple multiplication. Today's health care industry has a plethora of boards—hospital holding companies that layer boards on top of boards, with untrained boards instructing, or at least controlling, untrained subordinate boards. Thus, the ineffectualness of boards and their members permeates several layers and often multiplies itself. The situation is getting critical, I feel.

Interestingly, most hospital boards and their managements recognize the training problem. Every time I work with hospital boards, I hear board members complain about their inability to function as well as they wish. They talk about their skills shortcomings, their confusing commitments, their inability to relate to management and physicians, their disinclination to act boldly and decisively. They know they have problems. They quietly question the competence or commitment of fellow board members who are willing but weak. They sense that some people do not have the ability to be better board members and wonder how to get rid of them. All of these things and more are interrelated in something called boardsmanship.

The chapters ahead will deal with the ingredients that make for a successful hospital or health care corporation board. We will inquire into cause and commitment, because if board members aren't committed to the hospital's goals, everything else is academic. Then we will look at how to organize a board, and how to put together the best possible combination of people to form a strong, unified board. We will deal with the responsibilities of voluntary board members, both general and specific, and the symbiotic relationship of the board and management, as well as the quasi-partnerships of the board and the medical staff. And we will look at several ways that a hospital board can evaluate itself.

Building a Better Hospital Board is just a small book, and it won't answer every question you have. But it is a beginning. At least I hope it will give you a way to look at yourself as a board member and at the fascinating gestalt of your own voluntary board. I also hope it will inspire you to ask some questions. If you are willing to work at it, your own board can become better.

The result will be a more satisfactory experience for each of you as board members—and a stronger base for your organization. Aren't those outcomes worth some effort?

1.

Who Leads and Who Follows?

Boards of directors are interwoven into the fabric of our country's social and economic history. Certain small businesses may operate for a while as sole proprietorships and some select professional service firms can exist as partnerships, but the vast majority of businesses and service agencies are set up as corporations, with some form of board structure.

Why the corporate form of organization? For a simple reason: While the death of a sole proprietor automatically dissolves the business, and the departure for whatever reason of a partner necessitates reconstitution of the partnership, a corporation theoretically is set up for perpetual purposes. The corporation will outlive its founders, its management, and its board members. The corporate form also offers the greatest flexibility for growth, redeployment of assets, ownership change, and financial planning.

As the role of hospitals changes dramatically, so the corpo-

ration has changed and is changing. Any corporation in the
current health environment is confronted with many challenges—from other hospital competitors, from physician competitors, and from federal and state government policies. If you
choose to do business as a corporation, the laws of every state
require you to have a board of directors.

In for-profit corporations, the role of a board takes in four
broad areas:

— The board offers advice and counsel to management.
— The board serves as a court of last resort in controlling
  and disciplining management.
— The board serves in any crisis when management
  needs to be replaced or represented.
— Theoretically, at least, the board represents the
  shareholders.

From earliest times, hospital boards were composed of
volunteers. They were first called boards of managers, and
later boards of trustees. Today, board of directors is fast becoming the standard title. Trustees for many of our public
institutions were usually drawn from the community leaders in
banking, law, the clergy, or business. Their presence gave
immediate credibility to the new hospital enterprise. That was
important, for hospitals in the nineteenth and early twentieth
centuries did not typically show a favorable return on investment. An early board's first responsibility (seldom stated but
always understood) was to make up the deficit if any existed at
year's end.

In those early institutions, boards made most of the policy
and operating decisions because trained management was not
available. If you tried to state succinctly the purposes of an
early hospital board, they might be:

— To provide a facility in which health care services were
  available.
— To staff the facility with necessary personnel.

— To ensure adequate funding of the facility for the maintenance and perpetuation of the hospital.

That early trustee mentality came from the word *trust* itself. The trustee was holding something of value in trust—the hospital building, the patient rooms, the operating suites, the laboratories, and, later, the tradition itself. And the trustee held these for the community's benefit; not for their personal use, but for the greater good of their fellow men. Lofty purposes indeed, and as long as the hospital's credibility was unchallenged, that model was generally followed for several generations.

The most common title today—board of directors—carries a very different connotation. Directors, as a group, oversee a professional management team usually led by a person called president and chief executive officer (CEO). In that relationship, the professional manager knows more about the business and the industry trends than does the voluntary board. The board "directs" the chief executive, who acts as its representative to achieve the short-term goals and to accomplish the long-term mission.

As hospital corporations relate to other business organizations, such as financial institutions or large purchasers of health care services, the title of board of directors conveys an equal status. Use of the terms board of trustees, regents, or governors may imply subservient status in these business dealings. Throughout this book, I will refer to the governing body as the board of directors.

Where institutions were founded as private organizations by a church or a wealthy philanthropic citizen, the corporate charter or trust guided and directed the board in its governance of the organization. Some of those early trusts could not keep up with changing circumstances. For example, Mr. George Hermann's estate, when Houston was a city of less than 250,000 (in 1915), promised to provide *care for the needy of that city*. This great magnanimous gesture did not foresee the size of that city today with its population of several million people. If the trustees of such estates had not adjusted to the changing world, they would long ago have spent the institution out of business.

Hospitals and health care corporations of today must keep costs competitive to survive. Boards must act wisely if they are to perpetuate the corporation. Failure to adapt and change the organization may mean dissolution of the original trust. Maintaining its position requires that the organization take initiatives. This sort of pioneering drive takes leadership.

It's not easy in today's hospital to get a good answer to the question: Who leads the organization? Textbook theory and idealists in the 1950s maintained that most institutions were led by a beautifully balanced triad of board, management, and medical staff. But that balance is rare. In my experience, either a strong board chairperson pulls the medical staff and pushes management to achieve results, or a shrewd executive lets the board and medical staff feel they are responsible, while he or she supplies the goals, targets, and ideals. In a few select cases, the excellence of a single physician supplies the momentum and the board and management provide the physical and financial resources.

Every successful organization I have ever seen had a strong leader, an individual who claimed "ownership" of the institution's mission, purpose, or major program. It was usually easy to identify the benevolent giver, the driving force in the fundraising effort, the dreamer who kept everyone enthused about what the place could be, the political matchmaker who could compromise to get results.

Consider the for-profit enterprise. It doesn't start with a board of directors. Usually it starts with a strong person who has a dream involving a particular product or service. Sometimes a great product or service grows because the market conditions demand its success. Boards enter the picture later, after an enterprise seeks to borrow money and the financial institutions, venture capitalists, and outside shareholders demand a means to watch out for their investments.

Occasionally, a board will be formed at the outset of a new venture, and will consist of investors who have a personal interest in the success of the enterprise. Even in these cases, however, the board has no mistaken idea as to who is leading. The board has faith in the ability of the CEO to develop the new organization. It is there to monitor, audit, and advise. It may share the ownership, but the board stands aside and defers to the CEO's leadership.

Do you recall that most boards in the 1970s wrestled with the ideal of calling their top executive *president*? Today, it's the routine title. But a few years ago, boards argued that it was improper for a "newcomer" to have a title that connoted leadership and authority. Many boards were unwilling to share ownership and to delegate leadership to a professional manager. Until the 1960s, perhaps because of a shortage of trained, experienced health care executives, boards may have justifiably felt they had the primary leadership role. But for almost 20 years we've had a stream of well-trained people flowing from the nation's universities into health care. The problem may be in those institutions where the board still believes that it, rather than management, really leads.

When a board questions the title or authority of the top executive, it usually indicates how it views the organization. Such a board is not viewing the hospital as a business engaged in health care but rather as a social service agency of the community. This may be appropriate for tax-supported institutions that could not function without substantial economic assistance. On the other hand, many hospitals that were brought into being by tax revenue find themselves today being asked to compete as a business, to pay their own way, or to annually accumulate a financial surplus. Such hospital organizations, unlike the water department or streets and sanitation departments, do not have a monopoly. They are becoming market-driven and self-sustaining. Boards in such organizations need to update their view of the board's role vs. management's role.

As health care has become more and more complex, the board is less likely to be a *manager* of the corporation (as most corporate bylaws state) and more likely to be an *advisor* to a well-trained executive.

The question of who leads is philosophically interesting. Board members can range from those with a casual commitment to overly zealous types who really want to make managerial decisions (or at least strongly influence them by sitting in on all decisions). It's my view that the pure non-profit board model is inappropriate for today's health care enterprise. On the other hand, the for-profit board model is foreign and also offers little role modeling.

To describe the leadership equation, it might be best to look at *individual leadership*, demonstrated by the CEO, and *group governance*, as it relates both to volunteer boards and to their corporate counterparts in the for-profit business community.

Individual Leadership

In my experience as a professional search consultant, I've heard people say they want leadership when they are seeking a new CEO or other top executive. You could get the impression that leaders are the solution to any organization's problems. You conjure up images of knights who ride in to slay the dragons (or to eliminate the competitors) and rescue the princess (reputation, market share, bottom line, etc.), to the eternal gratitude of the masses.

What are the qualities that everyone desires when they use the term leadership? Characteristics of leaders in successful enterprises of any kind would be weighted differently by each of us and circumstances might also change the priority of the characteristics. Here's how various board members we've interviewed through the years have characterized leadership.

Leaders take initiative. They never simply describe problems to their boards—they also recommend a clear course of action. They anticipate problems and propose solutions, sense the need for action, and convincingly present an action plan. And they are not afraid to be criticized and questioned. They may insist that a board take their recommendations or they will exercise the ultimate initiative and resign. Such leaders are as valuable as gold.

Boards frequently lament a lack of initiative on the part of their CEOs. Many fail to understand they may cause the problem by not demanding recommendations and solutions. Still others insist on involving themselves so deeply in operational issues that they cultivate an ingratiating type who is content to let the whole board do his or her job.

Leaders visualize a place for their organization in the future, regardless of changes and trends impossible to see. They don't wait for a government blueprint or a guarantee of what the world will be like in 1995. They know that if they provide the best service, with the best people, meeting documented—not imaginary—needs, they will not wilt before competition or regulations. They can give a board, a medical staff, an employee group, and a community something to work for and strive toward. They can give an "I have a dream" speech and they can inspire.

I've known several CEOs who had this vision. One in particular walked into a hospital after major board resignations and medical staff wars with a plan. His enthusiasm was conveyed with energy that inspired creativity among his staff, belief by board members, and hope among physicians. Leaders have dreams and they can make people understand and believe them. Boards need courage to hire such visionaries.

Leaders help others learn and grow. They realize that for an organization to move and grow, its people must learn and grow. They want board members who get better and a management team made up not of "bucket carriers," but of associates who can and will challenge them. They provide a climate that nurtures risk-taking and allows mistakes. They encourage and reward managers who take initiative and get results. They want people around them with values, people who want to grow.

All eyes are focused on the CEO, for he or she is a role model. If a CEO is indifferent about basic values—showing common courtesies, respecting moral values, or providing quality service—who can trust the CEO in other areas? If a

CEO can articulate a strategy of service it is beneficial; *practicing* what he or she preaches is invaluable to team building.

Hospital organizations tend to be bureaucratic and political. People who are hired are often pressured to conform. It is the rare CEO who hires people who will break the rules or push to the outer limits of their responsibility—all for the sake of results. Those who create a climate for personal growth among their subordinates realize that the organization will grow in direct proportion to individual development.

Only the CEO can create this climate, but the CEO is hired by the board. Most boards hire based on consensus; if the board is willing to grow by the choice it makes, the ripple effect will follow.

Leaders delegate responsibility without exceeding the abilities of the people around them. They bring out the best in people to the advantage of both the person and the organization. They encourage growth by constantly challenging people. They perceive one of their major responsibilities as enhancing the organization's human resources.

Managing people requires patience and wisdom. Excellent CEOs, like coaches on athletic teams, get the best from each person and mold the total effort into organizational excellence. Leaders who are able to synthesize are able to discuss, debate, even argue, but finally reach positive agreements. Is it easy? No. But this trait can be cultivated.

Leaders follow established channels in their organization, but they are aware of informal channels as well. They deal positively and have all their cards on the table. They don't undercut their organization structure at random because that would undercut people they need to live and work with every day. They set an example for their board and their subordinates that will preserve the organization structure.

Organization structure is designed to increase organizational effectiveness. CEOs who treat their boards, medical staffs, and employee groups as political constituencies develop an *us* and *them* atmosphere. Boards that want leaders will need to express questions, concerns, and feelings directly to the CEO. Healthy leaders communicate their feelings and concerns to staff members and board members, to create a positive climate.

Leaders articulate a value system that helps subordinates carry out the corporate mission. They realize that lower-level personnel may lack the perspective to see in the long term. They realize that people will respond to worthwhile, honorable goals if they are reminded, reinforced, and reaffirmed.

A leader who values people will show it by rewarding the best performers. A leader who values quality service will know when to stop competing on price. A leader who knows the power of wisdom and truth will not rationalize until political outcomes replace corporate mission.

Leaders are attentive to people who want help, information, affirmation, or correction. They are always able to find time to listen to an employee, to question a board member's wishes, or to hear physicians with an idea. They know how to seek out complainers and critics to let them fully unload and unburden their negative thoughts, and when to take remedial action if warranted. They learn the wisdom of the old adage, "The Lord gave people only one mouth but two ears— for a reason."

People truly are an organization's greatest resource. Most of the nation's most successful CEOs are products of administrative residencies. That training period early in their career gave them a coach, a critic, a listener who helped them grow. How many CEOs are showing that same personal interest in tomorrow's leaders? Developing people is not busywork or incidental. It may be the biggest responsibility a leader will ever encounter.

Leaders get things done. They set goals that are achievable and then realize them. They make commitments and keep them.

They promise results and they deliver. They understand that the measure of leadership is organizational accomplishment.

Search committee members I've interviewed always express their preference for people who get things done. CEOs who combine knowledge and sensitivity with dreams and drive will get things done. These people have a sense of urgency that the bureaucrats don't have. They don't want merely to survive and keep their job—they want the organization to prosper.

The bottom line to this list of traits that define leadership is that *no one has them all*. Styles will vary from one organization to the next. It would be a classic mistake to assume that any one person can possess all these characteristics.

My experience indicates that boards seldom select the strongest leader, for fear that he or she will challenge the board. Remember, most board members feel the hospital is *their* hospital. Any board that wishes to break the old traditions will find it difficult.

Group Governance

A board is a group of people acting in concert. It takes on a unique social character because of the mix of its members, their environment, and how they react to one another. Each board develops its own role models, traditions, habits, opinions, and views. The overall style will run from conservative to liberal, with most groups leaning to the conservative. The group process is usually complex, hard for people to describe or capsulize, and frequently the group may be contradictory or unpredictable.

All persons have slightly different views on everything. When board actions are described as unanimous, frequently one strong, articulate spokesperson has actually made the group seem unified.

Voluntary boards are usually gatherings of well-intentioned people who must learn to trust one another. Strong personalities frequently must learn to harness their individualism. The more the group interacts, the more the board develops its own sense of character. Every time old members rotate off a board and new members replace them, the character changes slightly.

Can a group lead? In actual practice, it is more likely to govern—a subtle but important distinction. In my experience, successful boards have a majority of people who possess these governance traits:

— A desire to cooperate toward achieving the institution's goals. People who can state in positive form what they favor are infinitely better than strong-willed individuals who can tell you what they oppose.

— The ability to think objectively, logically, analytically. At every board or committee meeting, management presents proposals that require review and approval. Members must be able to analyze logically both sides of any question.

— The ability to speak clearly to the issues. Those board members who are able to crystallize the thoughts of the group into a summary statement or compromise solution are priceless.

— An open-minded attitude and respect for others. Sounds simple enough, but many groups cannot provide direction because the members can't get agreement among themselves on priorities or objectives. When people have mutual respect and trust for one another, easy give-and-take will prevail.

— An appreciation of the group process, but not to the point of paralysis. People must learn that discussion, input, and analysis are necessary, but sooner or later action must be taken or meetings become "sound and fury, signifying nothing."

Truly, board members develop esprit de corps after they have worked together a while and accomplished some significant results through their group effort. Just as in team sports, team success breeds trust and mutual respect.

Group governance in for-profit business organizations is

rare, usually seen only in more mature organizations that have a strong tradition: When the organization wins, everyone wins. Boards in public corporations are selected with much greater care than in voluntary organizations. Personalities of new board members are analyzed to complement—not confront— the chairperson or CEO.

The effective hospital board understands that its role is theoretically to direct the organization, but that in practice a competent CEO is hired to formulate programs, policies, and strategies and to chart both long- and short-term results. When the board starts to actively engage in decisions, it is demonstrating a lack of faith in the CEO's leadership. Those boards that are dominated by a chairperson who wants to run both the board and the hospital don't readily tolerate a second strong individual.

The group may lead in a leadership crisis, such as bridging the gap between CEOs, but this is clearly a temporary role. Leadership of organizations as complex as today's hospitals requires persons experienced and trained in institutional management. Effective leaders understand the business they are in. They understand the economics, competitive strategies, programming, facilities, and personnel issues. Successfully managing today's multimillion dollar hospital enterprise is a job for a professional manager.

While the bylaws may charge the board with a responsibility to "manage" or even "direct" the business of the corporation, the board does not manage in a hands-on, operational sense.

Here's the best description I've ever seen of this concept:*

> The word *manage* comes from the French word for "to control," as in dressage—the control of a powerful, well-trained, high-spirited horse through subtle, barely visible signals. The analogy is appropriate for the relationship between a board and management, and specifically, its chief executive. If the board wants to lead an organization, it has to go afoot, as in leading a horse. If it

---

*Reprinted, by permission of the publisher, from "Leadership and the Board of Directors," Jeanne M. Lynch, *Management Review*, August 1985, p. 28, ©1985 American Management Association, New York.

loses the power, it loses the pace and the drive of a competent executive body; it might as well be leading a dray horse of a management, without spirit, initiative, or independence. Invariably, when a board tries to run a company, that's the kind of management it gets.

On the other hand, when a board lets a chief executive lead without the appropriate controls, it runs the risk of a runaway, a poor performance, or a management that wanders off to graze— looking for greener pastures through diversification, or serving their own interests rather than those of the corporation and its owners.

There is a middle course, which I have seen in organizations with active and effective boards. One that gives the appearance that the chief executive is providing all the leadership, but has, in reality, the subtle signals and ultimate control come from the board. It is not an easy relationship to achieve. It takes time, it takes effort, it takes mutual independence, and, as in the case of the dressage horse and rider, it takes mutual respect.

The question—who leads?—is therefore answered. It is management's job to lead. It is the board's job to be supportive, to establish a current mission and the policies by which management will implement plans and programs to carry out the organizational mission. Boards that insist on dabbling in the minutiae will want managers as their chief executives, not leaders. The question—who follows?—is also answered. Board, employees, and medical staff will follow a leader who leads.

New board members frequently ask, "What does this board do and what are my responsibilities?" They are not only concerned with the legal responsibilities but they are really asking, "Who is in charge; who runs this show?" The confusion over board and management responsibilities is a serious one.

Any board that has a discussion on leadership every two or three years will not be wasting its time. Legitimate questions from either the CEO or the board can be dealt with. When boards bury their feelings they are fueling future fires of dissension. Periodic clarification of leadership roles protects against power struggles.

When a board must question its chief executive's ability to lead, it lacks the trust and respect to keep that individual. If the board finds itself doing management's job, the organization may lack a leader. There is plenty of meaningful work in any hospital for both the chief executive and the board. In the following pages, the board's job will become very clear; and the job will be infinitely easier if the board employs a leader.

2.

Cause and Commitment

Think back to the first day someone asked you to be on the board. Perhaps it was a telephone conversation, a luncheon, or a chance meeting at the country club. What was your first thought? Probably, "I wonder if I can be of any help." Your next thought might have been, "But I know little about what exactly a hospital does, and I know practically nothing about the health care industry." When you finally spoke, you probably said something like, "What would I have to do?"

Awkward, wasn't it? You were being recruited for an obviously prestigious position about which you knew little or nothing by someone who may not have known much more about it than you. How much better it would have been had the board member handed you the hospital's mission statement and given you a chance to respond to it. If you had job specifications and a job description, that would have been even better.

Belief in the institution's cause is the most essential element that any board member brings to the table. Lukewarm commitment by a director is dangerous. People who are intellectually challenged or who find board service interesting are fine, but boards need a majority who believe in the organization's cause, who are excited about its reason for being, its need to succeed, to grow, to expand. When directors have that zeal, the organization can succeed against sometimes frightening odds. If this element is absent in the enterprise, it is only a matter of time until we hear discussions about market saturation and the downside of product or service cycles. The next steps are exploring a merger, contract management, or calling in the auctioneer.

But there can't be commitment if there isn't any *cause*—a clear, official statement of the organization's goals, usually called the mission.

Corporate Purpose and Mission

A hospital must have a driving purpose. Its board must know why the hospital exists and then make decisions based on an understanding of and commitment to that purpose. It should be expressed formally in a mission statement to which the board can continually refer, like a ship's captain refers to a chart.

Without a mission statement, a hospital tends to wander aimlessly, not knowing where it wants to go as an institution, unable to plan sensibly. A hospital without a mission statement is one governed by the Alice-in-Wonderland principle. When Alice conceded that she didn't know which way she wanted to go, the caterpillar on the mushroom consoled her by saying, "Then it really won't make any difference which way you walk." Luckily, Alice survived her adventure. Hospitals that don't know where they're going usually don't.

The rudder of purpose—cause and commitment—will steer a health care corporation through many turbulent seas of competition and societal change. Without such a rudder, the corporation will surely run off course and perhaps ultimately even destroy itself.

There is no other board duty as critical to organizational success as ensuring that the organization has a current mission statement. This is a fundamental expression of *why* the organization exists, *how* it will function, and *who* (the markets) it will serve. It provides focus and answers to both board and management during any crisis.

Recently, I spoke to a board at its annual retreat and learned that half of the people on the board did not know there was a mission statement for the organization! Those who knew of its existence did not remember when it was last revised. Amazing, pathetic—but true!

A focused mission is like the coherent light of a laser beam. Some organizations seeking growth might visualize their mission as a flashlight beam, broadening out as it reaches ahead, hoping that somewhere in the future the goals will be touched upon. However, the best mission is like a laser, specifically highlighting a market segment or program.

Or, you can think of the mission as the hospital's lens. With this powerful lens, a hospital can concentrate its buildings, its equipment, its people, its tradition, and its community support on accomplishing what would otherwise be impossible. Remember, you can start a forest fire with just a magnifying lens and a dry leaf. At the most elemental level, the mission is about direction—which way and how you point your resources.

If directors state a hospital's mission too broadly, they defeat themselves. Goals that are too lofty become unrealistic pipe dreams. Unrealistic goals tend to be quickly forgotten.

It wasn't too long ago that few hospitals positioned themselves in the marketplace to provide ordinary-person care or care for the middle-income family. Every hospital acted as if it were a university teaching center or a junior Sloan-Kettering. They were all going to be "the best," an unrealistic mission for a hospital with a small endowment and no teaching faculty. Nevertheless, these hospitals acquired expensive new equipment and initiated programs with little regard to whether the programs would pay for themselves. In these cases, faulty mission statements undoubtedly contributed to the high cost of hospital care.

Directors are expected to be visionaries. While a clear mission statement allows directors to audit management's progress on approved plans and programs, it must be revised to adapt to changing environments. Most boards fail in this area and, by default, they allow management and the medical staff to plan major shifts in strategy.

While the prior examples suggest the problems for organizations with no mission statement, too broad a mission, or one that's unrealistic, another situation is far more common—every board member having his or her own idea as to why the hospital exists.

For example, in a board seminar I conducted on this subject, 7 members of an 11-member board had the following answers to the question, "Why does the hospital exist?"

President of a local manufacturing company: "To provide the lowest health care costs in the area."

President of the medical staff: "To provide the physicians with a place to bring their patients."

President of a local college: "To provide health care services and training for health care professionals and paraprofessionals."

Local attorney: "To provide jobs while providing a community service."

President of the hospital: "To provide health-related services for an enlarging market at the most favorable return on investment."

Retired bank chairperson: "To provide health care for citizens of our community that is of the highest quality."

Board chairperson of the hospital: "To build a health care corporation that meets the market's need for services."

Until that group agrees on a mission, everyone will discuss each issue with a hidden agenda. They will each look at any program, problem, or opportunity in relation to how it affects *their* concept of why the hospital exists. That boardroom will sound more like a city council than a corporation.

Mission Statement Strengthens the Board

The mission statement makes the board stronger in the following ways:

Creates a strong board. The wrong way to nominate board members is to make a list of prominent people who might like to serve on the board and then approach each one to offer an invitation. This recruitment method is not likely to yield a strongly committed board.

The right way to choose a board is to make a list of the areas of expertise needed to direct the organization toward its goals, identify individuals who have the needed experience, and recruit them. But this nomination method requires a specific, realistic mission statement and a current strategic plan.

Unless a director knows where the hospital is headed and is committed to carrying out that mission, there is a risk—a probability, in fact—that the new director will try to impose his or her predispositions on the hospital. Anyone who joins a hospital board without a commitment to the hospital's mission is likely to bring ideas to the boardroom that may cause the organization to wander off course.

Provides a driving force for success. Achieving the mission statement becomes the motivation to serve. It is the main payoff for service. In effect, the nominating committee says, "We want you to take time away from your family and your work; we want you to assume potential legal liability; we want you to take on problems that seem unsolvable; we want you to embroil yourself in public issues that will make you unpopular with some of your friends—and we want you to do it *for free*—all because you believe in our cause."

A hospital's board of directors must have the faith and zeal of a band of revolutionaries. With that faith, anything is possible. If board members believe, money shortages mean nothing; the board will somehow raise it. Building deficiencies mean nothing; the board will build what has to be built. Staff inadequacies are only temporary; the board will soon attract and pay for whatever staff is necessary. A believing board will always find a way.

Rekindles zeal. It's not difficult to be zealous when you're building a new plant or remodeling an older physical facility, is it? The mission is easy to focus on with the help of an architectural rendering.

The further away a board drifts from the original zeal that gave birth to the facility, the closer the hospital gets to extinction. That early zeal must be constantly rekindled, albeit with different fuel. Through constant care and redefinition of the mission statement, however, and continual broadcasting, hospital board members can remain as excited about the organization's purpose as they were the day the doors were opened for the first time.

Nations sing national anthems before sports events, lodges recite creeds, and religions hold revival meeting to renew the faith. How does a hospital board maintain its zeal? It does it by reviewing and revising the hospital's mission statement *each year*, and communicating that mission as often as possible to the hospital's audience.

Public corporations publish annual reports that tell shareholders their goals and explain how each goal is achieved. Hospitals, in far too many cases, publish no annual report and therefore do not explain what they stand for, what they've accomplished, and what they hope to accomplish next. Probably not one restructured hospital in ten has run a full-page ad in its local papers or published an annual report to clearly state what it hoped to achieve in its last fiscal year.

No matter what the message and the mission are, they really can't be stated too often. A mission that becomes familiar to the entire community is one that is likely to be accomplished and accepted.

There are many ways to fire up the board. One example is a 15-minute presentation at the beginning of each board meeting, turning the spotlight on some unit, function, department, specialist, or area of the hospital—to dramatize how the hospital's mission is being fulfilled.

Focuses resources. A mission statement focuses the resources of a hospital by acting as a benchmark against which the board measures all of the hospital's programs and services. If a mission statement says that the hospital will provide health care for the citizens of Danville, Illinois, for example, and management proposes that the directors approve the purchase of a hospital over 200 miles away in New Buffalo, Michigan, the mission statement helps the board eliminate that idea from discussion rather quickly. Of course, expanding a market may be desirable to create a referral base from an outlying area. In that case, the board should modify its mission statement to include growth and expansion as goals.

Take the case of a physician who wishes to do some rather esoteric research, far afield from the hospital's mission. With a mission statement as a standard, such research expenditures can be nipped in the bud. It's just not the business the hospital is in. Or, suppose someone offers the hospital an opportunity to buy a laboratory, a cemetery, a gymnasium, an ambulance company, or a helicopter service. The mission statement serves as the primary standard against which these opportunities should be measured. It asks the question: Is this where the resources should be expended?

A mission statement provides *protection* against many new ideas, programs, and services. A mission statement is like the Constitution, and a board of directors is like the Supreme Court. Anything that comes before the court must pass the test of whether it is constitutional.

Evaluates management. If the primary function of a hospital board is to direct the hospital toward accomplishment of its mission, and the CEO turns that direction into action, then the board should evaluate the CEO on the extent to which the mission has been accomplished or advanced in a given period.

How does a board do this? If each year the board relates the management team's goals and objectives to the organization's mission, it becomes a simple process. Every member of management should understand how he or she is helping the institution achieve its mission. Astute board members learn to question programs and projects that may be of interest to management but are not essential to corporate purposes.

A later chapter on evaluating CEO performance comments in greater detail on this process. We may simply say here that the corporate mission is a good yardstick by which to judge management accomplishments.

Helps determine when to hold or fold. A mission statement can tell a hospital whether or not to continue in business. The board can look at the mission statement and ask itself whether it feels enough enthusiasm to carry on with that mission. Any organization should go out of existence when the board no longer believes there is a reason for being. The hospital plant may not be burned out, but the board could be. It could be tired of recruiting physicians, facing regulatory agencies, financial problems, quality assurance, and all the rest. There may be a point at which it bails out and invites someone in to manage the hospital.

Suppose, for example, the hospital's original constituency has moved away. It was created to care for a specific, definable group—German Jews in a borough of New York. When the hospital was founded in 1890, immigrants could not find Jewish physicians to help them, because those physicians were not allowed to practice in existing hospitals. Nor did most hospitals serve kosher food. So the immigrants got together and a hospital came into existence. But times changed. Jewish physicians, often the grandsons and granddaughters of those same immigrants, are now welcome on the staff of any hospital in the borough. Moreover, most of the children and grandchildren of the Jewish immigrants have moved away. The neighborhood is now predominantly Puerto Rican. And so, the board faces a hold-or-fold decision.

At that point, the board should scrutinize its mission statement and weigh it against the situation. Bailing out to the suburbs looks promising. But wait a minute! The German Jews in the suburbs can go to any hospital they want, so what's the point of recreating a Jewish hospital somewhere else? Meanwhile, where will the community's Puerto Ricans go? Now, we have a real test of board resolve, and a key example of the function of the mission. Should the board unload the hospital because the mission it was created to serve no longer exists, or is the true mission of the hospital to serve the *neighborhood*, regardless of who lives in it?

Suppose the board interprets its mission as serving a defined constituency and therefore decides to hotfoot it to the suburbs. Does its mission allow it to walk away? Twenty years ago, maybe; today, that's not an option. The responsible way to withdraw from an old neighborhood, and the way truest to the spirit of the original mission of the hospital, is to relocate gradually and to provide assistance to the institution that remains behind.

Sometimes, holding is the best course. I recall eating one of the finest meals of my life in Fort Wayne, Indiana, in a restaurant that was the former site of a Dairy Queen drive-in. The owner had seen his market moving; competition from other fast food chains was all around. He could have closed down and sold the land to someone else. Instead, he converted the site to a small, exquisite restaurant, which now draws its clientele from a four-state area.

Not all situations have tidy endings. Sometimes, the best choice may honestly be to close the doors. On the other hand, when commitment is extraordinarily strong, the board may be able to bring a seemingly terminal institution back to health. Only the board involved can decide if the mission is worth fighting for—and whether it still has the wherewithal for that fight.

Provides a platform for telling the hospital's story. Once while driving to a client meeting, I happened to hear a listener call-in program on a country music radio station and the subject was health care, of all things. The program was a revelation. Caller after caller expressed anger at hospitals, each one telling a personal horror story. It occurred to me that hospitals do little or nothing to correct these negative public impressions. The folks in advertising call it "copy platform," a way of presenting the organization in a unified, positive fashion.

While hospitals busy themselves with restructuring, reorganizing, and responding to legislation, they may forget to communicate their reason for being. Most hospitals leave this onerous task to professional groups: "Let the hospital association do it, that's what we pay dues for." But hospital associations can only do so much, and they certainly can't deal with the specific problems of every one of their hospital members. Besides, it is a hospital's responsibility to explain itself to the public. It is not a task that can be passed on or passed over.

The mission statement should be the underlying theme of every hospital communications campaign. The story should be told over and over again in a variety of ways, with reference to numerous credible sources. Over time, if the creative campaign is put together properly, the "soul" of the hospital will come through to the general public.

Keeping the Mission Fresh

A mission statement should spell out the hospital's general philosophy, describe its reason for being, and define the objectives the hospital seeks to achieve. The mission statement should be flexible, so that it can be changed when new medical practices, a changing constituency, or new laws and regulations develop. Three sample mission statements appear in Appendix A.

When reviewing a hospital mission statement, the board should ask basic questions: Why are we in business? What is our position? What opportunities do we face? Such questions may seem self-evident to board members who are business people; perhaps that is why they don't ask them.

Board members must accept that many of the questions

facing them will not have clear-cut answers. For example: Is our cause worthwhile? Is our goal right? Is it realistic? Are we doing all we can to pursue our goal? Time is another critical element in this examination. Directors must ask: Are we moving too quickly or too slowly? Are we ahead of the market or are we behind it? Are we leading our competitors or following them?

Addressing the question of competition and relating it to the mission statement is especially important in today's "hospital-eat-hospital" survival contest. For many hospital boards, this is a difficult problem to contemplate. In all likelihood, their mission was established when there was no hint of competition, and no thought of hospitals vying with one another and other health care entities for the patronage of patients. If the hospital was the only one in a town or neighborhood, it therefore received all of the community's ill and injured, all of its professional support, all of its emotional support. The hospital held a monopoly. But towns grew, and other hospitals appeared with overlapping service areas and redundant programs. More important, patients became consumers, choosy about their health care providers. This upheaval in the health care environment will continue into the foreseeable future and, thus, hospital boards must learn to reset their compasses periodically.

Hospital boards should begin the process of refreshing their mission statements by deciding what they are *for*. Fundamental? You bet! Do hospital boards do it? Generally not. Most boards do not know what they are *for*, but only what they are *against*. This may be a reason why so many hospital boards are reluctant to re-examine the question of their mission. Yet they must, if their hospitals are to survive and succeed and prosper.

What is the major competition for each of the services the institution provides? Does the mission statement suggest that the organization will try to expand? Even at the expense of putting other competitors out of business? What if the competition in key areas includes select members of the institution's medical staff? Boards have been sitting on the fence for some time on these key questions. In today's racetrack atmosphere there will be winners, losers, and drop-outs. And the mission's appropriateness will be one of the major determinants of that success or failure.

Perhaps when you were asked to be on your board you didn't get a chance to study the organization's mission. It's entirely possible that you didn't understand what a job on the board would involve. But ask yourself if you want the next person who serves with you on the board to have the advantage of understanding the organization's purpose. And ask yourself if, by selecting people who know the cause and believe in it, you'll be helping to make your board better.

3.

Toward an Elite Board

Elite units in the military are composed of the best people, people selected for the right reasons who are willing to serve for the right purposes. Specifications are developed and studiously adhered to, and because the specifications are elite, the best people compete to serve with the very best.

The nation's first astronauts were selected in this way, as we all saw in the film and book, *The Right Stuff*. They had to have extensive flight experience, proper education and training, superior personal character, and a willingness to serve. They might be killed or they might flunk out but they had to be better than average even to apply. While the risks are somewhat different, I'm suggesting that the process is applicable to board selection.

An elite board is composed of objectively selected individuals who have the collective know-how and desire to direct the organization toward fulfillment of its mission. Hospital boards should be small, efficient, elite cadres of people who have been screened for certain qualifications, especially experience at governance. Such a group is not easy to assemble. Nor is it easy to hold the group together once assembled. Today there are fewer people who can be valid candidates for hospital boards, and many of those are either unwilling to commit for the length of time required of a hospital director, or have other matters on which they would rather spend their time and energy. Yet, if you want your hospital or health care corporation to succeed, you must create such a group.

A result of modern lifestyles is that fewer people are available to be hospital directors or, for that matter, directors of any kind of voluntary organization. Families today often have two or more working members; one of them might have been, in another day, an outstanding candidate for hospital board membership. Today, they just don't have time. Instead of putting in hours every month as a volunteer director, some people spend their total energies working their way to the top of their companies or professions. Many of these upwardly mobile people will give time and energy to work on projects, but few are able to give what it takes, year in and year out, to be a good hospital board member.

To gain a rough idea of how the demand for board members exceeds the supply, assume that the average hospital board in America has nine members (a *most* conservative estimate) and that there are 6,000 hospitals in need of directors. That is 54,000 directors, and to find 54,000 you need to sift through 300,000 candidates. You would not be overly selective if you chose one of every six people you considered. Then, too, remember that hospitals are not the only organizations seeking board members. Staggering! Within the context of this enormous demand, place hospitals' needs for directors against a rapidly shrinking pool of potential candidates. The inference is obvious. Any hospital board that wishes to constitute itself as elite must invest substantially in locating and keeping good members.

How Directors Currently are Selected

Since the demand for directors is high and supplies of elite people are very low, boards need to devote more time to the process of finding and selecting directors. But historically, nomination committees have typically done little homework. A few names are dropped; often, that is all that is necessary for consideration. In appointive and elective boards, the process may be even worse. Smaller communities often rationalize their choice of people by concluding that their pool is smaller. Selection of directors, to put it kindly, is a fair muddle.

Most common is the *self-perpetuating* board—new members asked to serve by those already on the board. Terms of office vary from fixed, multiyear terms to invitations to serve for life. Self-perpetuating boards today are likely to offer back-to-back terms to keep capable people a reasonable length of time.

Other boards are selected by an *appointment* process: a governor, mayor, city council, or bishop appoints people to serve, usually for a stated period of time. These boards have special problems because the appointers may not use a logical method of selection. Many times I've worked with appointed boards that desperately needed a person experienced in finance or legal matters. One group asked the mayor to appoint a person skilled in financial affairs and capable of chairing the finance committee, and got a retired postal worker, instead! Another group requested an attorney because the board's deliberations raised legal questions, and the city manager appointed an inactive elementary school teacher! Such boards need to publicly request the specific help they need so that appointments by public officials will at least be made in the public eye.

Then there are *elected* boards. People actually do campaign for the office of hospital board member. Some boards have overlapping terms of office, while others have all seats vacant at the same time. These latter boards usually become political and are least likely to understand their role in relation to management. I know of one physician board member who was inspired to campaign for a board seat when his admitting privileges were revoked for 30 days for late medical charts. He also induced a fellow physician to run for the board, and the two created occasional havoc in that boardroom.

Nominating committees do the preliminary selection work on most self-perpetuating boards, but they often lack a written set of qualifications. Without a method of screening candidates, they may look for anyone willing to serve. I have listened to multimillion dollar health care corporation board chairpersons ask their members, "Who do you know who might make a good board member?" without any specific reference to qualifications.

For every other position in the hospital or any business organization we would have a position description and position qualifications. Failure to follow those basic steps would be considered questionable business practice. Yet, it happens in the boardroom all the time.

A Screening Process

A logical way to improve selection is to define as objectively as possible the characteristics you are looking for and then seek people who have them. Think of the process as a funnel with a number of filters inside. Just below the widest part of the funnel is a coarse filter, and just below that is a slightly finer one, and then a series of increasingly finer filters. If you poured all of your candidates for board membership into the funnel, and if you selected your filters properly, those who passed all the way to the bottom of the funnel would be the people you want as hospital board members. Your specifications are the filters to help you get the elite people you really want.

Filter A: Experience. Get a staff person to visit the local chamber of commerce and systematically go through the board membership of every organization, including churches. Compile a list of all the people in town who currently serve on voluntary boards. Those are the people who, along with their out-of-town counterparts, would pass through the filter at the top of the funnel. They have gained the experience—some good, some bad—of getting things done as a member of a group on a board. It is invaluable, unique experience. You should not consider for membership of your board anyone who has not had recent experience on some other board. Board experience is fundamental.

It may not seem quite fair to exploit the boards of other organizations for the benefit of your hospital board, but the hospital business is competitive in more ways than one. You want the best. You will get the best if you identify people with voluntary board experience. Look at it this way: Service on other boards is merely preparation for the hospital board member's difficult task.

To make the first cut for the hospital board team, then, candidates must pass through the first filter—experience at governance.

Filter B: Achievement. The next important requirement is achievement. The person you're considering should be an outstanding contractor, or the best attorney in town. Business people should not be struggling to survive, beholden to every banker and politician around. You want the cream, the people who have risen to the top. These are the people who can best resist pressure. And you can be sure they'll have plenty to resist.

Professional achievement will give the board candidate a base of credibility with other board members and the community at large. People who have not experienced substantial professional achievement may view their role on the board incorrectly. Some may see the board position as that of power broker while others may view a board seat as their crowning professional achievement.

Filter C: Occupation and skills. Having screened down to

achievers experienced at governance who are personally secure, you should now consider occupation as a qualifier. Every hospital board needs different skills at different times. If the hospital is considering a new form of organization, the board might find management consulting skills useful. At other times, the situation may require legal, financial, communication, marketing, or even political skills.

Keep in mind that one of the functions of a hospital director is to provide advice and consultation to fellow board members as well as to the CEO. If the hospital has embarked on an extensive program of diversification, the CEO would undoubtedly find it helpful to have a board member with some understanding of the fields into which the hospital is diversifying. If the hospital is trying to overcome a serious image problem, the CEO might like to be able to turn to a public relations professional, or an executive who has had intensive public affairs experience. If the hospital has invested heavily in new programs that must attract new customers, the CEO might be well served by the presence of a marketing expert on the board.

How a hospital board constructs its skills filters will depend greatly on its strategic plan. A board should anticipate the kinds of skills that need to be represented on the board, so that they will be available to the CEO.

Filter D: Team play ability. Being on a board is a team sport. No matter how outstanding, how bright, or how desirable in other respects—if a person is incapable of subordinating himself or herself to the board, that person will never make an effective board member, and should therefore be screened out.

This requirement unfortunately eliminates some of the community's entrepreneurs. As a rule, entrepreneurs prefer to do things themselves, rather than in concert with others. The primary oracle they consult is their intuition. They are accustomed to action, but while boards need to act much more readily than they have in the past, they need to act as one. A board is a choir in which each member sings a part to produce a single sound. It is a blending of talents. This is not to say that the board members should be everlastingly agreeable. Far from it. But after all the debate and discussion, after all the give-and-take, the board should be able to decide as one, pulling together as a team.

Filter E: Affluence. Traditionally, the hospital director assured the fiscal health of the institution. The boards of many hospitals used to be groups of the wealthiest people in town, people who could financially contribute to the hospital and influence their friends to do likewise. The function of hospital boards has expanded well beyond the purely fiscal, but there is still reason to have wealth represented on the board. Many wealthy people have a high degree of social consciousness and the time to devote to worthwhile causes. While they may not have the intensely independent spirit of their forebears, they do have the financial ability to go their own way, without worrying too much about community pressures. They tend to have great status in the community. Their family or business name is well known. They have clout with the right people. Assuming they have the other qualifications, people of means can be excellent hospital board members.

Filter F: Positive associations. A highly positive feeling about the hospital enhances a person's ability to be a good director. Such a person might have had a parent, child, or a best friend whose health problem was resolved by the hospital. Such a person usually feels good about health care institutions generally and particularly the hospital where that service was provided. Avoid at all costs the person with negative associations. He or she can damage the hospital, perhaps permanently.

A positive attitude in the boardroom, on the other hand, uplifts the entire board. I once ran into a director who did wonders for the board simply by expressing his attitude in the local paper. Here's a paraphrase of it: "I've lived in this town most of my life. I have been to the hospital at least four or five times. All my children were born there. The hospital is an integral part of the community and has been doing good things for us for years. When I was asked to serve on the hospital board, I wanted to do nothing more than to help the hospital be as good to other people as it has been to me and my family." Find someone like him for your board.

Filter G: Personal qualities. A director's personal qualities will enhance the performance of the board. The most important of these is *intelligence*. Hospitals are arguably the most complex businesses in America today. Their problems are not for dull minds.

Board members should also possess and demonstrate *compassion*. The business of hospitals is not cold or hard, although it must seem so at times to the people delinquent in paying their hospital bills. Hospitals are literally in the business of caring. Board members must feel for patients, and be sympathetic to their problems. Patients are not only customers, they are people who need help.

Board members should also be *good listeners*. They should not bring personal agendas to the board table, but rather open minds. They should be willing to grow in the job. There are no overnight wonders in the hospital board room; it takes time to become an effective member of the board of directors.

Underlying all other personal qualities are *high moral/ ethical standards*. A hospital board member is the Caesar's wife of the community, above reproach. If there is such a thing as a community pillar, that pillar should be the hospital director.

Filter H: Objectivity. The objectivity standard must apply to all board members. No one on the board should represent a specific constituency. Each board member should be an at-large member, representing no one and everyone. Elected board members sometimes make poor directors because they try to grapple with public opinion regardless of organizational needs. Any time a director forsakes the mission to serve another purpose, the board becomes political and the organization suffers.

This requirement of objectivity can be nettlesome, because it will screen out many of those traditionally thought to be the likeliest candidates for board membership. Consider, for example, that a local business executive might stand to gain from decisions made in the hospital boardroom regarding insurance. Hospitals usually are the biggest businesses in a given community, because they have the largest payroll, and they often have substantial endowment funds to be invested. Can a banker be objective about how those monies are invested? Some can and some can't; some will pass through the screen of objectivity and some will not.

Filter I: Staying power. Until recently, non-profit hospital boards often perpetuated themselves. When a director completed one term, the board simply gave him or her another. Few directors ever resigned voluntarily. By the 1970s, though, self-perpetuation had fallen into disfavor, and the favored buzzword of the boardroom was "turnover." I must admit it was one of mine, too. I feel differently now. Today, I'm in favor of self-perpetuation—assuming qualified directors who understand their responsibilities and their accountability, assuming continuing director training, and assuming a zealous commitment to the hospital's mission.

I've reversed my position because the health care business has become too complex for amateurs. Some of the health care programs evolving today will take years to complete, and will require the attention of directors who are willing to commit themselves to the long haul. I find that it takes, conservatively, three to four years for a hospital director to begin to understand what's going on, and a few more for real skill to develop.

I don't condone the Rip van Winkles of the boardroom, but greater emphasis should be placed on recruiting and keeping people who are willing to listen, to learn, to change, to grow. Directors who have served five to seven years have just begun to be valuable. It's a waste to lose that perspective, wisdom, and insight if they are performing well.

Filter J: Receptivity to training. After all candidates have been identified, screened, and admitted to the hospital board, they must be trained. Training is so important, in fact, that I advocate a minimum amount of annual training for hospital directors be written right into the hospital's bylaws.

For a board to act wisely, it must be made up of people who can keep up with what might be called state-of-the-art boardmanship. A person who is too busy to attend retreats for board development or seminars is too busy to be on your board. Board members must accept the need to develop their ability more rapidly than simply by living another year in the position. Hospital bylaws should require all board members to attend two or three training sessions per year. Training is the board's own quality assurance tool.

Most boards could be strengthened immediately if they established both fiscal and time budgets for board development. I believe that a board today must spend a minimum of $500 per member on board development. One hospital in Ohio allocates its per capita board development as follows:

Magazine subscriptions for each member $ 50.00
Books for each member $ 50.00
Guest speakers two or three times a year $100.00
Registration for one in-house retreat $300.00

Keeping Track of Candidates

The entire process of selecting board members can be facilitated by a simple form. In any business, applicants fill out employment applications that ask for information on their education, training, experience, interests, and skills. That form is kept on file so that even if the person is not currently available, he or she can be contacted again when a position is open. With the scarcity of qualified board members, we can hardly afford to do less.

Here is a sample form that you can adapt to create a similar bank of potential board members. Prepare one for each board candidate so that the nominations committee can better understand the individual, and keep it on file for the future if he or she is qualified but cannot serve immediately.

Sample Board Member Information Form

Date _____

Name _____

Office Address _____

Home Address _____

Home Phone _____   Office Phone _____

Current title or occupation _____

---

1. Candidate's Previous Board Experience:

   A) Organization _____

   Sales volume or budget size _____

   Tenure _____

   Committees _____

   B) Organization _____

   Sales volume or budget size _____

   Tenure _____

   Committees _____

   C) Organization _____

Sales volume or budget size _____

Tenure _____

Committees _____

2. Candidate's Areas of Expertise: _____

_____

_____

3. Special Health Information Related to Candidate:
   Consider any health problems that affected parents, spouse,
   children, or close relative.

   _____

   _____

   _____

4. Candidate's Philanthropic Interests:
   What causes, political parties, or charities does this individual
   support?

   _____

   _____

   _____

5. Candidate's School or Educational Affiliations:
   What schools did this person attend or support?

   _____

   _____

   _____

6. Candidate's Hobbies and Interests:

_____

_____

_____

Source: Witt Associates Inc.

Data for this form should be accumulated by the board committee or its staff person, with the exception of item 3, special health information. The information and data gathered will help the committee decide whom they will pursue for positions on the board. Keeping files and records on all potential board candidates for the future is also extremely helpful.

After a committee has determined that a board candidate is of interest to them, a face-to-face visit will be necessary to determine if the person understands the corporate mission and is willing to accept the responsibility of the board work at that particular institution.

The person making the first visit will be selling and persuading. Many people are tempted to turn you down because they feel they'll be giving more than they are able to get. If you can sell it as an opportunity for a person to learn, grow, and contribute, you'll have greater success.

It is essential to leave an information package with prospects for board membership. This might include the following:

— Mission statement of the corporation.

— Position description of the board of directors.

— Latest annual report.

— Latest year-end financial report.

— Organization chart of the corporation.

— List of current board members.

— Newsletters and brochures that describe the organization's services.

The purpose of the first meeting is to sell the institution and its mission to the potential board member. But it is also critical that this be considered a "screening meeting" for both parties. The prospect may not wish to be a candidate for the board, or the board may decide another person is better able to help the board at present. In such cases, that prospect may be called upon at another time.

Don't select board members because of their prestige, organizational position, or net worth. If these people don't share a belief in the cause of the organization and have the time to commit to board work, they should not be asked to serve.

Recruiting an elite group of people to serve on a board is a year-round process. Searching for new corporate directors has caused many boards in recent years to engage executive search consultants for this task. Hospital boards that want to improve will find the development process frustrated unless the caliber of persons they seek is truly elite. Somebody said, "You can't make a silk purse out of a sow's ear, unless you start with a silk pig."

4.

The Mechanics of Board Organization

No matter how good its members, a hospital board needs structure to effectively carry out its mission. Thus, the elite board members discussed in the previous chapter must organize themselves to respond to needs quickly and decisively. The size of the board, the mix of its people, the types of committees it creates, the direction of the board, the monitoring of the board, and other issues of mechanics are all important to the board's effectiveness.

Boards tend to be shaped by a variety of factors. Strategists and planners recommend organizational structures that provide a logical framework for the relationships between board members, management, and the medical staff. But the people involved determine the real structure. Some boards simply select a chairperson and let that person organize the board as he or she sees fit. Others just borrow the constitution and bylaws from some other hospital, and sometimes boards accept these as if they were graven in stone. Many CEOs recommend periodic changes in board organization to reflect changing needs and marketplace realities.

Time as an Organizing Principle

What a hospital board can accomplish depends, assuming qualified board members, on the amount of time board members have to carry out their responsibilities and how that time is apportioned. The organization of a board should be based on the amount of time available from board members for board-as-a-whole activities and for more specialized board activities. That is, figure out what has to be done, determine how much time is available, and divide one into another to discern the structure of the board.

Most people who serve on hospital boards have no idea of how much time they must spend in meetings. Nor do they realize that the time they spend in meetings is directly and proportionally related to the amount of time required to staff the board and its subdivisions. I've seen hospital boards with so many committees that the entire management staff became bogged down preparing papers for meetings, attending meetings, and writing minutes. These can be high-priced when you consider that the minute-writer may be paid a six-figure salary!

After board members understand and accept the hospital's purpose, they should know exactly how much time they are expected to devote. That commitment cannot be open-ended. Potential board members shy away from such blank checks for time. In fact, many qualified people refuse to serve on hospital boards, saying, "I can't afford the time," often before they know how much time will be required.

Discussing what is a reasonable amount of time each month for board activity is worthwhile, especially if it helps the board to focus on how much or how little time is being spent on each area.

A hospital board must indicate how much time its members should contribute to the board overall, to the executive committee, and to standing or ad hoc committees. This should not be loosely indicated. The board should lay out the year and decide how much time it expects of its members—12 hours a month, for example—and provide a breakdown of how that time will be spent. For example, board meetings of two to three hours plus committee sessions of two hours might ideally mean four to five direct hours per month and another three to four hours preparing and discussing issues between meetings. I say monthly here because that is how most hospitals presently divide up time, but as you will shortly discover, I strongly believe that most hospitals should begin to divide their years by 4 instead of 12.

The true test of a board's organization is whether the board can find the optimal time required of board members, and divide that time optimally to achieve hospital goals. A board can require too much time of its members. When board members spend, say, 20 hours per month working for the hospital, they are spending too much time, unless there is some kind of emergency. Sometimes, a board member's willingness to spend excessive time in board activities is interpreted as deep commitment. In reality, it is a sign that he or she has crossed the line from being a director of the hospital into being a manager of the hospital. This is a board member who is more involved in operations than is desirable.

Frequency of Meetings

To attract the best people to the board, and to make the best use of their time, hospitals should meet less frequently and pack much more into the meetings—as most colleges and for-profit corporations do. In so doing, hospital boards can add people to their membership from virtually anywhere in the world. By meeting monthly, hospital boards deny themselves much talent that might otherwise be available. Outstanding people cannot always make monthly meetings, but they may be available on a quarterly basis.

To attract the best people, I suggest that hospital board

meetings should be held quarterly, rather than monthly, or at the most, six times per year—every other month.

Quarterly meetings do not reduce the amount of time a director must devote to the hospital. It will merely be *rearranged*. Instead of three-hour meetings once a month, boards can meet for two days every three months. On the first day, committees or task forces of the board can meet to intensively review management's staff work, discuss their own concerns, meet with experts for consultation, and generally conduct the specialized work of the board. On the second day, the entire board can meet for four hours or so to consider the conclusions of the committees. Changing from a monthly to a quarterly meeting schedule might also jar those boards who have become too involved in managing hospital activities into streamlining their roles and returning to a directing mode.

This approach to board organization has important implications, not only for the kind of people who serve on boards, but for the size of hospital boards and the way they subdivide themselves.

Compensation for Directors

A modern hospital board might want to include among its membership out-of-towners who can contribute to the board in special ways. Then it might be possible to consider paying directors a stipend for the time they spend serving the hospital. The board members of industrial corporations are paid for their service—why not hospital directors? Those who can afford to serve and those who have time to serve are only part of the universe of good people.

At the risk of touching on a sacred issue, I would like to question why hospitals do not pay board members. This issue is always buried before it receives any honest discussion. I submit that the following are reasons to consider compensation of board members:

— An organization could be much more selective in recruiting people if it could move outside its immediate community.

— Experts in various functions and those with a knowledge of the industry could be sought.

— Retired health care professionals could serve as valuable members of boards, bringing all their years of perspective to the boardroom table.

— Committees could be composed to best deal with the policy issues being considered.

— Since all other members of the hospital leadership receive compensation, and incentive compensation as well, it would be only fair.

Many times in the past I've debated this issue but always with the professionals (hospital executives or physicians) and seldom before board groups. Many board groups consider it taboo, a despicable subject. But I would point out that less than 20 years ago all physicians took voluntary call in emergency rooms. Today, emergency room medicine is a recognized subspecialty. In many institutions, the voluntary chief of staff has been supplanted by a paid medical director. In both cases, institutions have strengthened their quality of service by paying for the services they need.

A word of caution: If boards consider compensation before they set standards of performance, they may get nothing for the money spent. But if they use compensation as part of improving overall governing board performance, it would be money well spent indeed.

Board Size

Most hospital boards are too bulky and unwieldy to react quickly enough to exploit opportunities. There's a historic context for this cumbersomeness. Prior to modern financing mechanisms, board members essentially underwrote the hospital. If the hospital ran in the red, board members made up the difference out of their own pockets. Thus, a $350,000 deficit for a ten-person board meant that each board member would write a check for $35,000 at the end of the fiscal year, or would raise that amount from friends of the hospital. To spread out this fiscal responsibility, boards simply added members. In time, boards of large hospitals frequently numbered more than 100 people.

Most hospital boards in America today could double, triple, or quadruple their effectiveness by losing some weight and becoming a fraction of their present size. If we assume that the average board of 12 with five to seven standing committees is appropriate, then ideal size projections are possible. Generally, smaller hospitals with revenues of $20 million or less should have boards of *no more than five to seven directors*. Larger hospitals, with revenues of $20 million to $100 million and more, should have boards of *no more than 15 directors*. That is the limit. No board, no matter how large the hospital, should have more than 15 members.

Now, I am aware of all the arguments for large boards. All aspects of the community must be represented on the board, some will say. Others argue that all of the monied interests of the community, especially old money, must be represented on the board against the inevitability of a fund-raising campaign. Still others caution that various constituencies of the hospital should be represented on the board: for example, the medical staff, the women's board, auxiliaries, the church, the city, ad infinitum. Nonsense! A hospital board is not a congress. It is an organization that audits management, a device designed to chart a course for a hospital and then to assure that the hospital management stays on course.

Pruning hospital boards to acceptable limits, of course, will cause pain. There is no painless way. Whenever a board member dies, retires, resigns, or moves out of town, simply pull his or her chair away from the board table, and don't replace it. Retire it. Not just the director, but the director's slot. Attrition may not be sufficient to take care of the problem of an oversized board, however. That may require bolder action. By decree, transform the executive committee of the board into the entire board. Then dissolve the old board or empower a committee to make selections for the new, smaller board.

Decreasing a board's size is the perfect focus for a two-day retreat to discuss board purpose, size, style, duty, discipline, and accountability. Most board members shy away from any direct attempt at downsizing to escape charges of power-grabbing and of placing leadership with the favored few. The fact is, courageous action of this sort is the stuff of which healthy, vigorous enterprises are made.

Balance and Mix

An elite board must not only be made up of the right people—sharp, bright, well-trained people who have a strong interest in the hospital's mission—but it must also be made up of different kinds of people in the right proportion. It must be heterogeneous, not homogeneous. To be strong, it must be an alloy, not pure metal. What's wrong with like-minded, like-talented, like-disposed people making up a board? Consider the following sequence of board requests.

— "Give me the facts."
— (Upon receipt of 147 pages of facts from management): "Give me a summary."
— (Three weeks later, after reading the sumary): "Give me your recommendations."
— (After hearing management's recommendations): "Let's call in a consultant."

Sound familiar? It should. It's the pattern most hospital boards follow. Why? Because they tend to be made up of the same *type* of person: the analytical, judgmental type who doesn't wish to gamble with community resources.

Judicious people are sought for board membership, and these people are often analytical by nature. And what could be more logical? After all, a hospital director should be wise, objective, fair, and capable of weighing facts and rendering a verdict based on them. The problem is that such a person judges often but acts rarely, or not at all. An elite hospital board needs some analytical types. But a board made up exclusively of analyzers invites paralysis. Such boards want action but seldom want to pioneer programs. Their favorite question is, "Who else has done this?" Their favorite comment is, "Let's wait until we have more information."

To get anything done, a board should be a rich mixture of tenure and skills and personalities. It should, for example, include a sprinkling of gutsy, intuitive types, to balance out the analyzers you can't do without.

Board committees also need a mix of people. In putting together a finance committee, for example, have someone on it with long tenure with the hospital board, someone with financial skills, someone with analytical skills, someone who relies on inspiration, someone who is a visionary, and someone who can serve as spokesperson. And keep in mind that these qualities are not mutually exclusive. A board member can have more than one.

Those of you who once belonged to fraternities or sororities may remember how assiduously the rush committee applied itself to recruiting pledges who would give the house a balance. A few scholars: but not too many, or you'd have an egghead house. A few varsity athletes: but not too many, or you'd be known as a jock house. A few musicians and artistic types, but not enough to be known as a cultural house.

You won't have a healthy mix when one person controls the board. An organization I once visited had an attorney on the board who was the power behind the scenes for three reasons. He was on a retainer as a salaried attorney to the religious order that operated the hospital. He was chairman of the board for a bank whose president was the hospital board chairperson, and as a former board chair himself, he was chairman of the nominating committee. You can just imagine the problems that arise in boards like that, in which power is so centralized.

Although hospital directorships should not be lifetime appointments, they should last at least 10 years, and preferably

15. Given the great competition that exists today for good hospital directors, hospital boards should invest heavily in selecting and training their directors. That human investment should be treated like any other hospital investment in human resources, and be kept productive as long as possible.

Public Corporate Committees and Hospital Committees

Most public corporations have six standard committees:

— Audit
— Executive
— Finance
— Strategy or corporate objectives
— Personnel/succession
— Compensation

Functions vary from one board to another but the audit committee is set up to work directly with the corporate audit firm and its internal auditor. Its basic responsibility is to verify the credibility of financial statements and internal controls. Executive committees are set up to move quickly and process matters of immediate concern that cannot be dealt with by the full board meeting. Finance committees occur in corporations with large capital budgets or recurring external financings to ensure that management's use of corporate financial resources is prudent.

Committees that oversee corporate strategy and objectives focus on broad, long-term issues. This type of committee keeps refocusing the corporate mission, financial objectives, and corporate criteria for success. Personnel/human resources or succession committees ensure that the organization's policies and practices provide a continuing stream of highly motivated, trained people to keep the business prosperous. Compensation committees in public corporations understand that key executives need special rewards. They must remain competitive but not "give away the store."

In contrast, hospitals function with many committees, but the most common are:

— Finance

— Executive

— Nominations

— Planning

— Joint conference

— Quality assurance

Finance committees monitor monthly budget variances and approve major capital expenditures and revisions in either revenues or expenses. Executive committees are also set up to move more quickly than the full board, which requires more lead time to convene. Nominating committees are responsible for finding the next group of directors and officers that will serve the organization. Long-range or strategic planning committees try to focus on the future facilities, program financing, and corporate mission of the organization.

Joint conference committees are unique to this industry. Usually they are composed of the officers of the board and officers of the medical staff organization or some combination of this sort. The theoretical intent of this committee is to guarantee that structure does not prevent communication. If the medical staff leadership needs to question the board on an issue, this committee allows the communication to take place within an organized structure. Conversely, if the board needs to question the medical staff, it may also do so. This committee prevents small "end runs" around the structure by either board or medical staff members. A worst-case scenario would be one in which a problem arises and no one resolves the issue.

Finally, the quality assurance committee has recently emerged as a key group that monitors the quality of medical care provided. This committee reviews physician and hospital practices as well as policies that may need reinforcement or revision.

Divisions of the Board

The principle of economy that applies to the size of the board should also be applied to committees. Board effectiveness can depend upon limiting their number, size, and longevity.

There is an overgrowth of hospital committees in America that needs tending. They are the health care version of kudzu. At many hospitals, some committees don't function and everyone knows it. They exist only because "they always have."

Generally, committees of the board should be replaced by ad hoc groups set up to deal with specific problems within a certain period. That is, all committees of the board, by whatever name they are called, should be temporary. They should go out of existence after a prescribed period, usually the end of a fiscal year or the conclusion of a phase or a project.

Instead of having standing (or *leaning*!) committees, create a separate task force for each committee chore. A bonus: You'll be able to add talented people to the task force who are not board members, people who can bring particular skills or interests to the task.

The advantages to using ad hoc committees that function like the sunset legislation in some states are:

— These groups function with a greater sense of urgency to get the job done.

— People have a feeling of involvement in a current issue.

— Better people may serve, knowing the assignment has a beginning and an end.

— Involvement by non-board members becomes practical. The committee can serve to test the potential of future board members.

— Ad hoc groups tend to have a better definition of their
tasks than standing committees. At times, the standing
committees seem to build agendas to fill the time allot-
ted to them.

To Be or Not to Be a Holding Company

Should a hospital become a holding company, just because
it is the fashion? The answer lies in what the board has decided
the hospital's objectives should be. If the board is ready to slug
it out in the marketplace not only for consumers but for new
and perhaps different kinds of businesses, then a hospital holding company organization might be appropriate. If not, a holding company is a waste of time, energy, and money. And who
can spare those?

Unless a board's appetite for competition and conquest is
very strong, cold feet become the rule about three to five years
after reorganization. Board members begin to ask: Why?
Where are the payoffs? What's the return on investment? Competition is fine for the consumers, but it costs the competitors.
Many boards members are interested in a hospital but they're a
little hazy on what a new-ventures, for-profit health corporation is all about.

Structure precedes strategy when establishing boards in
non-profit organizations. Boards are formed first, before the
organization. In contrast, in most business enterprises there is
first an idea, a concept, or a product. Next, there are people
who believe in the idea with all their hearts. They work,
scheme, dream, build, shape, until the success of their concept
causes an organization to form. After the organization is
formed and capital is sought, a board is formed to oversee
management. The board in fact may be demanded by the bank
or venture capitalists to watch their investment.

Most new ventures require quick decisions. Too much governance before there is anything to govern will create organization and structure before there is a real reason for being. First
decide your mission, then organize to accomplish it, pick a

winner to run it, and get out of his or her way. Be tough in monitoring the progress and demand results that are tied to deadlines.

Board Tenure

In retreats and seminars I'm often asked, "How long should I stay on the board?" As your board term ends, ask yourself these simple questions. They'll help to sort things out.

— Do I still feel a zealous enthusiasm for the mission of this organization and its programs?

— Do I feel that this group of board members is effective?

— Are there people more qualified to serve than me?

— Is there another board on which I'd rather serve or another public service I'd rather perform?

— What strength or skill do I bring to the board that can't be replaced?

Information Needs of the Board

Somewhere between being buried in a blizzard of paper and being kept totally in the dark is the right amount of information necessary for a board to do its job. The basic ingredients for an effective information system are:

— Minutes of previous meeting.

— Agenda for each meeting and advance distribution of all material prior to the meeting.

— Financial statements.

— Periodic special reports by the CEO or key industry spokespersons.

— Special presentations by key members of management or the medical staff.

At least once every three years a board should evaluate how well its regular and special information needs are being met, and tell the CEO the results of that evaluation. If changes in board membership result in requests for more information in a different format, this should be discussed. A frequently whispered concern of board members is that they don't get the proper information or don't get it in time. Why whisper? Open the topic up within the context of a discussion on board organization, and get what you want.

Self-Criticism Improves Board Mechanics

Tradition and boilerplate bylaws frequently determine how a board is organized. That should not be the case. Board members should be constantly critical of their own efforts to ensure that time spent in board activities is productive, not merely ceremonial.

Boards today are showing a willingness to critique their own work efforts. Whenever this is done, it leads to a new learning experience for all members of the board. A board willing to look at its own organization and make the tough decisions to change is a board that is learning and growing. Until and unless boards begin paying stipends for service, that growth experience may be the greatest reward available.

5.

The Board's Responsibilities

No question is discussed and debated more often than "What is the role of the board?" New board members ask, management frequently seeks clarification, and physicians question how the board views itself. It is certainly a valid question. It is necessary that all the board members understand their job.

The extent of board participation in management runs on a continuum from casual indifference to excessive involvement. Boards are involved in management prerogatives for three reasons: They lack confidence in management's ability or decisions; they simply desire to "run the show"; or they are ambiguous about what the board's role should be. If a board fails to understand its role clearly it will flounder in minutiae while policy issues are avoided.

Everyone has a different concept of what a board's job really involves. Decision-making in hospital boardrooms involves a panoramic range of technical, ethical, financial, medical, regulatory, and logistical fields of knowledge. Board acts are corporate and are arrived at through a group process. To make sure board members have a current and correct perception of their roles, something concrete needs to be created: a written job description.

Position Descriptions

For many years I have advocated written position descriptions for the board and written statements of purpose for all committees and task forces. If a hospital organization can prepare position descriptions for clerks, technicians, managers, and executives, there is no excuse for failing to define the board's responsibilities.

There are three excellent reasons according to modern human resource experience for defining position responsibility:

Recruitment. A written description will not only help the nomination committee focus on the right talent, but will also let potential recruits know what is expected of them if they join the board. Most of today's board members would consider that a luxury, but in fact it's a necessity.

Orientation. A position description provides a point-by-point look at a director's role, allowing a new board member to ask more informed questions and to become more quickly oriented. Boards must accept responsibility for their own orientation and self-perpetuation.

Appraisal and assessment. A hot board topic is performance evaluation of boards. What better way to start than with a clear position description? Spell out what you want, and you can expect people to perform. It also offers the chairperson a specific tool with which to reorient an errant member and clarify what the preferred performance outcome is.

The added benefits of a position description may be clarification of lines of authority, better self-understanding by all the participants, and a more clearly focused use of everyone's talents.

Preparation of the position description, whether done by a consultant, a committee of the board staffed by management, or by the board at a retreat, has as much positive benefit as the end product. When board members have to think about and discuss their responsibilities, they gain an understanding of and appreciation for their position. Some boards will try to copy another board's description, but every board has a unique mix of skills, personalities, and prejudices. The other guy's shoe just won't fit.

General Board Functions

Here's a list of general duties, responsibilities, and powers—a composite document, drawn from various board seminars I've conducted. No single board could use all of these, but the list will help any board that is trying to formulate a position description.

Establishing a mission. If there already is one, keep it in focus. If conditions dictate a change, revise the mission and purpose of the organization. This means a regular revision of strategic plans will be necessary. A board may look to the CEO and management staff for recommendations or they may seek periodic assistance from consultants to make certain the mission is current and meaningful and that progress toward it can be measured. Mission statements are best developed around the answers to some very basic questions:

— What business are we in?
— What is our position relative to our competitors in each of our major markets?
— What future opportunities do we have?
— Where are we going in the next three to five years and how will we judge our progress?
— What should we be doing to ensure our future success?

Selecting and evaluating the CEO. This is the most commonly understood duty of a board. But spell it out anyway. Seldom clearly explained in policy or in procedure form, it involves a four-part process: defining specifications, interviewing candidates to assess their skills, attracting the candidate of choice through persuasive skills and diplomacy, and evaluating the CEO as he or she fits into the new role.

Working well with the CEO. Some boards feel they have a responsibility to work successfully with the person they hire. Other groups apparently feel that the CEO must relate to them. Some boards compete with the CEO for leadership and management of the organization.

The ultimate success of any hospital organization depends on a board and CEO who are able to work well together—not merely to tolerate one another, but to have enough mutual respect so there may even be dynamic tension. This means the relationship is never without annoying moments. The key is for both parties to keep investing in the relationship by honestly stating their feelings.

Granting medical staff privileges. This is a duty unique to hospital boards, one that historically has been misunderstood. During the 1970s, the push for quality assurance programs helped boards see this responsibility more clearly. However, few boards understand that the composition of a hospital's medical staff is not an accident. Failing to add new specialties to the medical staff has seriously limited many institutions. The right mix seldom just happens; it is caused by a board that understands this responsibility. Some board members believe that because a medical staff is "self-governing" it means that the board has no authority over the physicians. Not true! It must be accepted and clearly understood that the board has the authority and responsibility to oversee its medical staff.

Fiduciary responsibility. Boards in non-profit hospitals make decisions and act for the greater good of the community. Boards generally understand that they control corporate assets, and they appreciate their liability in the newly emerging health care corporation. They are acting as trustees for the organization's assets.

Specific Board Duties

While these vary from one organization to the next, a discussion of many of the familiar duties may be helpful. Here is a sampling of duties representative of many institutions:

Effective organization. This is the real key to unlocking the talents of all the board members. The successful board organizes around its members' talents and expertise to assure optimum performance. Most boards inherit a structure and work with it; few realize that organizing around talents and interests will assure maximum input by everyone.

Corporate values. The board sets the tone for the basic values of the entire enterprise. A strong conflict-of-interest statement sends a clear message to everyone involved. A well-defined mission statement also tells employees, physicians, and the public what the board believes, and what it holds sacred. Policies concerning indigent care, employee relations, or public relations will also reflect values.

Policy development. A board that finds itself rehashing the same problems over and over needs to look at policy development, to cover recurring situations in which uniformity of action is desirable, efficient, and effective. It is management's duty to administer the programs of the institution, but it will be done more effectively when guided by board policy.

Many directors are sincerely concerned about how to influence direction, initiate new programs, and generally get the ball rolling. The problem is, they are trying to please all the major players, and too often clear policy decisions are not made. Directors need to commit the organization, management, and medical staff to specific policies.

The more a board recognizes its responsibility to focus the institution's policies and objectives for all major aspects of the business, the more successful it becomes. Directors must *direct*, and they do it with policies.

CEO performance evaluation. The board hires and fires the CEO. It also should regularly review how the CEO performs and communicate its assessment of that performance to the CEO. Few hospital boards have a written policy and procedure for assessing the CEO. Criteria are seldom formally established and goals are not mutually agreed upon. In addition, few boards have a written executive compensation policy complete with current salary ranges. How does your board handle this part of its job? Could this procedure be strengthened or improved?

Solvency responsibility. The board, working with management, must keep the hospital solvent. Every worthwhile hospital has encountered financial crisis at some time—often because it took on the financial risk of starting a special program that was financially unwise, but morally impossible to walk away from. Current trends point toward hospitals becoming "cash-and-carry" operations, where only economically feasible programs with adequate return on investment are maintained. But the responsibility to meet community needs will always raise social concerns in the mind of the committed board member.

Today's hospital boards wrestle with the issue of indigent care. They agonize between providing services to people who cannot pay, or refusing them services. In a business sense, every board has a fiduciary responsibility to do what is economically prudent. In a moral sense, some boards accept responsibility to find the funds for charity, but they will define the amount and accept their share within limits.

Board influence. A credible board member can promote the programs of the institution. Board members are conduits to the community generally and to the financial community particularly. Members with political influence can use it judiciously, to advance the organization's cause. An occasional problem is the well-meaning but unwanted help some board members give without having sought full board approval.

As health care has come under greater regulatory pressures, hospitals are finding that boards have political responsibilities as well. Directors should understand that using their influence is a big part of their job, although it is often left unstated until the need arises.

Institutional objectives. A board must make certain that the annual objectives are being met. When there is failure, the objectives need to be reviewed or the methods used to develop them need to be changed. Many boards assume that the organization's mission is obvious and that management's goals are its own business. Both parties must sign off on the goals and financial plans and name the priorities on each list. This prevents management from pursuing those goals that are easiest or of greatest personal interest. The board that fails to establish priorities has little right to complain about a lack of institutional progress.

Acceptance of supervisory responsibility. After the mission and the corporate value system are determined, all decisions and actions must be consistent with the cause. The policies enacted can either pinpoint what the board wants management to achieve or they can be hazy platitudes that leave both the board and management in doubt. Too many hospitals exist from year to year, considering survival an accomplishment. If the organization is *not* growing and succeeding, the board should look first in the mirror and then at management.

Preparation. Athletes must work hard and practice to perform at their best. Boards are like athletic teams. For board meetings to be productive, members need to prepare, accepting whatever work or study is necessary. No board member can be a spectator.

Attendance at meetings. This duty sounds simple enough, but it should always be spelled out in position descriptions. It's equally important for regular board and committee meetings and for educational and developmental meetings. When a board assessment process is used, this factor will get its proper consideration.

When an organization makes every effort to develop its board by providing books, magazine subscriptions, seminars, and retreats, it should get a fair return. Far too few boards require attendance at development sessions, so often members who most need the exposure may fail to get the message.

Assignments finished on time. This is essential to efficient board operations. Some board members mean well when they volunteer for an assignment, but they do not get the task done. The chairperson will want to consider a discussion with these individuals.

Confidential deliberations. Keeping all conversations private is a courtesy to fellow board members. If board members rush out after every meeting to tell family, friends, peers, or business and professional associates what the institution is thinking about, a business atmosphere becomes a political arena.

Failure to keep board meetings confidential ensures that few people will really speak their mind. If board members feel they'll be quoted or their votes will be discussed in public, the board's meeting will become a carefully rehearsed performance.

Positive contributions to board discussion. Some people serve on boards and are quiet, except to tell fellow members what they are against. Negative comments or questions asked in a meeting to embarrass management (especially when they could have been asked in advance, allowing proper data and information to be assembled) are in the best interest of no one.

Consultant activities. Many board members are sought for board membership because they have special expertise. Their assistance to the CEO and, with his or her approval, to other executives in the institution, is a valid duty. Wise CEOs learn to seek such counsel and advice. On the other hand, board members need to realize that unrequested advice may be given but the CEO reserves the right to select his or her own course of action. Rejecting advice does not make a CEO wrong; it may indicate that he or she is not afraid to make mistakes.

A working knowledge of hospital practices and health care trends. Acquiring this is the hardest duty for some members. Here is a short course that provides competency:

— Understand the statement of purpose of your committee.

— Read minutes for the last two years of the committee meeting to familiarize yourself with the issues.

— Have the board chairperson or CEO arrange visits with at least six board members from six different institutions who serve on similar committees to enlarge your perspectives.

During your first year's membership, ask for a list of periodicals and books to enlarge your perspective. Every board member should maintain a broad knowledge of hospitals and the health care system in our society. Too often, board members plead ignorance of issues. Most people begin with little knowledge but it is their responsibility to learn more.

Directors on any board should be alert to new programs, services, and products. Long-range survival requires that the organization continually prepares for the future. A board should always be changing, adapting, growing, and keeping management on its toes.

Avoidance of conflict of interest. Experience has shown that hospital boards need to develop a firm, clear statement on this matter, signed by each member. Legal and financial services are the two most frequently abused areas.

Position Descriptions

The following sample position description outlines the basic responsibilities of a board of directors. Board job descriptions for two hospitals are given in Appendix B.

Sample Position Description for the Hospital Board of Directors

General Functions

The hospital board of directors' basic responsibilities are to:

— Establish and maintain the organization's mission.

— Act as trustee for the assets and investments of the shareholders or owners in the non-profit corporation.

— Select, advise, and audit the CEO.

— Grant physicians staff privileges and ensure that quality medical care is provided.

— Provide broad direction for the affairs of the hospital and ensure the development and growth of the institution's services.

Specific Duties

The hospital board members' specific duties are to:

— Prepare for board and committee meetings by whatever study and preparatory work are necessary to deliberate intelligently with co-directors.

— Attend meetings of the board and committee appointments.

— Execute board assignments on time.

— Maintain confidentiality and security regarding hospital information.

— Contribute positively to board discussions, assisting the board in reaching conclusions.

— Serve as a consultant to the CEO and, with his or her approval, to others in the organization.

— Acquire a working knowledge of those functional activities for which he or she has committee assignments.

— Develop a broad knowledge of today's hospitals and future trends in health care.

— Be alert to new program opportunities and assist the organization on specific programs when requested.

— Avoid interference in hospital operations.

— Avoid conflict of interest whenever an issue arises, and abstain from board discussions when matters in which he or she has a personal interest are being considered.

Source: Witt Associates Inc.

The concept of a position description for the board may seem elementary, but with so many people rotating on and off hospital boards, it becomes a necessity. Any board that spends enough time clarifying its own role will more clearly appreciate management's need to lead and manage. More important, board members will see that establishing the mission, strategies, and policies to run a corporation is a fulfilling, rewarding job. Boards with a well-conceived position description will also appreciate the need to develop and improve themselves as a vital first step in overall organizational effectiveness.

6.

Evaluation of the Board of Directors

Board evaluation must be a threatening concept, because few institutions adopt an evaluation policy without considerable debate. Many business and community leaders feel that, as volunteers, they'll do the best they can—but who wants to invite criticism for their voluntary effort? Yet the process of evaluation can be a positive learning experience. Self-criticism indicates high self-esteem and mental maturity.

In 1976, at the Maryland Hospital Association trustee seminar in Ocean City, I told the audience that although we audit the medical staff to assure quality, and we audit the management to assure its credibility, the board seems impervious to an audit. I said it's time that directors took their responsibilities as seriously as do management and the medical staff. Several years previously, I had argued at board retreats that the improvement of hospital boards must be tied to a director's position description and standards of performance. Today, although there is interest in the subject, too many boards and

CEOs are still looking for the perfect process—one that has been proven at 100 other organizations.

An overall evaluation of operations in a multidimensional business like a hospital is difficult, but not impossible. The most common problem seems to be establishing criteria or standards of performance. Judging by the small number of hospitals that have an effective board evaluation system, it's safe to speculate that boards may not have devoted sufficient energy, time, or resources to this subject.

Boards offer interesting examples of group dynamics. Individual directors legally have little or no authority; they must come together in a group. If we are to improve a board, we can either work on individual development needs or group development needs. All boards can be characterized by how they work together and react to one another.

It is always a learning experience for the new director to come to know the group mood. New directors view their fellow directors with varying degrees of skepticism. As they work with their fellow board members, they sense the roles that various members play. Every board needs to have people who play different roles. The roles range from creator/innovator to critic, from social conscience to pragmatic administrator. An evaluation procedure should help individuals and the group understand their strengths and weaknesses in these roles.

Any evaluation process, regardless of the method employed, will require that members of the group be honest and open and have basic respect for one another. If a board member can't help a fellow director conform to increase group effectiveness, the board misses experiencing its full potential. Whether the problem is a fellow director who talks too much or one who doesn't participate enough, that issue needs to be addressed. Failure to attend to these and other matters will eventually lower the team spirit of that board.

Benefits of Board Evaluation

These are some of the reasons why a board evaluation process is essential:

Clarify what directors expect of each other. People wonder whether their work in the boardroom is sufficient, proper, or adequate. Role clarification is essential if we expect effective performance. Under normal circumstances a board reports, as one board chairman stated, "only to God." For this reason, self-appraisal or some form of peer feedback is essential.

Many boards I've worked with had a board member or officer who was generally acknowledged to be acting in inappropriate ways but everyone avoided a confrontation. A mechanism must exist to release the pressures that build in groups when things are left unsaid. Whether people speak too little, too much, or too negatively, they can profit from knowing how they are perceived.

Review and renew the board's sense of purpose and mission. Without continual effort to renew board members' zeal, the organization will lose its momentum. Every opportunity to keep the board's interests fine-tuned is worth the effort. The less a board takes its heritage for granted, the less likely it is to sell the charter for mere dollars.

Any board that is willing to look critically at itself cannot function with an outdated mission. Improvement and growth will become more real to everyone associated with the institution when they see the board serve as a role model. Any organization that identifies its strengths and weaknesses at the governance level will stay eternally healthy. Those that only engage in finger-pointing and second-guessing of management and the medical staff set a poor example.

Develop agreement on specific priorities. Everyone may assume they know what management should do and what the board expects, but evaluation pinpoints any lack of clarity. When a board can't agree on its own objectives, it cannot give solid direction to management or hold management accountable for implementing policy.

A few boards I've known had chairpersons who constructed a "board objectives" plan annually, based on their fellow directors' assessments. The board must have deadlines and specific goals for its own improvement or it will drift. Good intentions remain exactly that—intentions.

Improve the effectiveness of board and committee meetings. In the evaluation process, board members may see that a written statement of purpose for committees will focus everyone's effort and improve meeting mechanics. The committee's performance can be improved significantly by cutting down on the number of meetings. Few boards have ever had seminars on this important subject but they spend 100 percent of their effort in meetings of one sort or another.

Help pinpoint organizational problems for remedial action. As a board reviews its organizational purpose, channels of communication, responsibilities, authority, and organizational structure, areas that cause problems are identified. The fundamental step in problem-solving is to define the problem.

Improve the composition of the board. An evaluation will highlight the need for specific expertise along with proper mixes for age, regional representation, and a variety of other factors. It will make the need for membership criteria more apparent to the board. Occasionally, after a board undergoes a self-evaluation, an individual board member will resign, realizing that his or her contribution was not what the board needed.

Heighten the quality of board information. As a board seeks to improve its performance the need for timely, adequate information becomes clear. Board members need to communicate with each other and with management regularly to assure that the advance information package is doing its job.

Develop future board training needs. As boards see where they are weak or lacking in information, they can literally form their own agenda for future board development sessions. One board I worked with in New Jersey discovered in the first year after its self-evaluation process that it needed to know more about three internal departments, and it selected two subjects for future outside speakers.

The Process

"How do we start the process?" Boards frequently get frustrated by the effort to pick the perfect process, but there isn't any one best method. The process usually begins with the establishment of a policy that clearly states the board's intentions.

Evaluation is not a project for one or two people on the board; the decision to self-evaluate must be made by everyone. Whatever method you use for the process, it will take time, energy, resources, and commitment. This is a sample evaluation policy statement adopted by one board:

> It shall be the policy of this board to evaluate at least biennially both individual board members and the total board, to improve board performance.

At the same time as this policy was adopted, the board discussed its commitment to the process. After a lengthy discussion the board decided to *require* participation. Some boards fail to take this step and they may engage in circular discussions that produce no definite result when some members do not commit themselves to the process.

Some boards appoint a committee to draft a list of evaluation criteria. Others have management and a board committee develop the initial list. Regardless of what factors are included, the list should change to reflect any change in board thinking. A board is not static and unchanging, but is rather a dynamic, complex, and often contrary group.

Once a policy is discussed and adopted by the board, the methodology—a timeline with dates and deadlines—is the next step.

There are two broad approaches to the methodology for an evaluation process. First, a consultant might come in to review board operations. Or second, a board might engage in some form of self-evaluation.

Consultant Evaluations

A progressive board will periodically call in objective consultants to help it examine the functioning of the total operation. These operations reviews are helpful to a new board or one that is overwhelmed by criticisms from every possible corner about the organization. These studies provide tangible proof that the board is exercising its supervisory function and not being a naive rubber stamp for management.

Any board could use that approach to evaluate its performance. Some members may not have the time, talent, or expertise to engage in self-evaluation, however. Use of a consultant has appeal for them. The consultant's final report is presented to the entire board and any corrective actions may be scheduled for the months or years ahead. Successful business organizations feel that this approach strengthens the board.

Self-Evaluation

Self-evaluation is the second alternative and of the numerous approaches that may be taken, I've personally observed the three below.

Standards of performance. The first assumes that to have evaluation, you'll need standards of performance. Therefore, board discussion is held on the subject, with a standard of performance for hospital boards of directors as the catalyst document. I've included a sample of a board of directors' standard of performance in this section of the chapter.

If the board discussion is led internally, a strong or opinionated chairman can turn this into a perfunctory checklist. The result may be that the board is deemed to be perfect in performance and awarded an "A" for effort and commitment. Hurray! End of project and process. But did you *gain* anything?

For a meaningful discussion, boards may wish to have every member give his or her impressions, questions, and comments. If these discussions are recorded, the leader may then draft a written report of all questions and suggestions grouped by subject matter and send a final report to all participants. This document becomes a "to-do" list for the board with appropriate direction given to management as decisions are made.

Responsibility for the format and feedback may be assigned to a board committee, but those responsible must have experience gathering data and preparing written reports. This is, therefore, most often a staff or consultant assignment. Few boards will have people with the three ingredients needed for this type of project: experience, time to devote to the project, and a strong belief in the validity of the concept.

The best starting point for developing evaluation criteria or standards of performance is the director's position description. If your board has not developed a position description, that may deserve first priority. The following "generic" standards of performance for a hospital board might help you get started.

Sample Board of Directors' Standards of Performance

The hospital board will be considered adequate with the accomplishment of the following tasks:

— There is a written mission statement, statement of purpose, or board policy that defines what the board does, and how, why, where, and when it is done.

— Short-range (annual) and long-range (three years or longer) goals and objectives have been established for the total organization.

— Action plans have been established in writing with assigned responsibilities for accomplishing the long-range objectives.

— There are current written position descriptions for the board of directors, the board chairperson, and the CEO.

— The board has hired a CEO in whom it has confidence and who it supports.

— The board has appropriate policies and procedures for evaluation of the CEO.

— The board has appropriate policies and procedures for evaluation of the total board and its individual members.

— The board has written personnel specifications for its membership and its officers.

— The board has an appropriate policy and procedure for recruitment of new members.

— The board has a quality assurance program to oversee and control the medical staff.

— All board and committee staff work is performed by staff or consultants.

— The board annually reviews a program for personnel development to ensure adequate succession in the first three tiers of management—the CEO and two levels below.

— The board has a required policy for personal development of its members.

Source: Witt Associates Inc.

These standards are not intended to be all-inclusive. They are intended to help any board group stimulate discussion on the broad subject of standards of performance for boards of directors.

Please note that the first statement says any board that performs the tasks on this list of standards is *adequate*. Any standard that is too general can be more focused and any standard that is too complex for your particular board can be simplified. Be especially sensitive to adding standards that may have special significance for your group. Religious institutions may wish to include standards on values, for example.

When a standard is agreed upon—i.e., "The board has an appropriate policy and procedure for recruitment of new members," ask additional questions of each member.

— If there is a policy, do all board members know the procedure?

— Are all members satisfied that the procedure is up-to-date, practical, and appropriate?

— If clarification or revision is necessary, who will do it and when?

— Does the procedure produce the desired results?

Self-rating evaluation. A second method of self-evaluation is self-rating. Board members examine their own performance and competence. The ratings are then summarized and tabulated. If the majority rate themselves weak in certain areas, it's probably a safe bet that more time and educational effort need to be expended. The results again are a springboard to discussion.

Results of evaluation discussions are clearly an opportunity for decisions and actions. Failure to act, change, or remedy problems breeds an attitude problem among board members. If, for example, a board member indicates that his or her expertise is not being used, it will be vital to address that issue before the seeds of discontent are sown. Discussion of the self-ratings involves exploring the extremely high or low ratings to see why there is a problem or how perfection is achieved. The factors in a self-rating can always include issues that relate to decisions the board is currently making. It is important to keep these discussions focused on board operations and performance rather than on particular problem-solving.

The discussion leader for this type of session must be objective. The person with an understanding of many hospital boards will be helpful. Professors, consultants, or association executives can play such a role provided they are from outside the immediate geographic area.

This sample self-rating procedure will illustrate the questions that need to be asked in this type of evaluation.

Sample Directors' Self-Rating Procedure

You are being asked to rate your knowledge, performance, and understanding of the various criteria for members of the hospital board of directors. This is a simplified self-rating that each board member will complete for himself or herself. You need not sign or identify yourself unless you choose to do so.

All the ratings will be collected and tabulated and the results will be presented for full board discussion.

Most questions ask you to rate your level of information or knowledge on a low-high scale. If you rate your knowledge above average, for example, you might give yourself a 6, 7, or 8 or even higher on any given question. If you have doubts about any area or feel you're still learning, you might give yourself a 4, 3, or 2. Please be *candid* as you answer these questions about your own board knowledge.

A few questions may require brief comments. Use examples where it will help explain your comment.

1. Rate your knowledge of and familiarity with the organization on whose board you serve, regarding services, key personnel, corporate mission, goals, and objectives.

    1 ---- 2 ---- 3 ---- 4 ---- 5 ---- 6 ---- 7 ---- 8 ---- 9 ---- 10

2. How well do you understand your own responsibilities as a board member?

    1 ---- 2 ---- 3 ---- 4 ---- 5 ---- 6 ---- 7 ---- 8 ---- 9 ---- 10

3. Rate your relationship with the other directors.

    1 ---- 2 ---- 3 ---- 4 ---- 5 ---- 6 ---- 7 ---- 8 ---- 9 ---- 10

4. Rate your knowledge of the health care industry compared to other hospital board members nationwide.

    1 ---- 2 ---- 3 ---- 4 ---- 5 ---- 6 ---- 7 ---- 8 ---- 9 ---- 10

5. Rate your understanding of the hospital's competitors in the marketplace.

    1 ---- 2 ---- 3 ---- 4 ---- 5 ---- 6 ---- 7 ---- 8 ---- 9 ---- 10

6. Rate your involvement in the process of overseeing management recommendations for corporate goals and objectives.

Never 1 ---- 2 ---- 3 ---- 4 ---- 5 ---- 6 ---- 7 ---- 8 ---- 9 ---- 10 Always

7. Rate your knowledge of the hospital's physical facilities, for maintenance or replacement.

1 ---- 2 ---- 3 ---- 4 ---- 5 ---- 6 ---- 7 ---- 8 ---- 9 ---- 10

8. Rate your attendance at board and committee meetings.

1 ---- 2 ---- 3 ---- 4 ---- 5 ---- 6 ---- 7 ---- 8 ---- 9 ---- 10

9. Rate your participation in board meetings.

1 ---- 2 ---- 3 ---- 4 ---- 5 ---- 6 ---- 7 ---- 8 ---- 9 ---- 10

10. Rate your reading of minutes and other information prior to board and committee meetings.

Never 1 ---- 2 ---- 3 ---- 4 ---- 5 ---- 6 ---- 7 ---- 8 ---- 9 ---- 10 Always

11. Rate your willingness to keep board and committee discussions out of non-policy management and operating issues.

Never 1 ---- 2 ---- 3 ---- 4 ---- 5 ---- 6 ---- 7 ---- 8 ---- 9 ---- 10 Always

12. Are there any real or potential conflicts of interest in your service as a member or officer of the board?

Yes _____

No _____

Comments: _____

_____

_____

_____

13. Would you be willing to serve as chairperson of a committee or as a board officer?

Yes _____

No _____

Comments: _____

_____

_____

_____

14. What do you feel are your strongest areas of knowledge, experi-
    ence, and competence? (Mark all that apply.)

    _____ Advertising and promotion

    _____ Consumer wants and habits

    _____ Employee relations

    _____ Energy

    _____ Engineering

    _____ Environmental issues

    _____ Financial management

    _____ Governmental affairs (local)

    _____ Governmental affairs (state and national)

    _____ Investments

    _____ Legal

    _____ Management information systems

    _____ Materials management

    _____ Medicine

    _____ Marketing

    _____ New product or service introduction

    _____ Planning

    _____ Real estate

    _____ Technology

15. Are there any areas of expertise that the board or CEO are not
    properly using to get the greatest benefit from your board
    service?

    Yes _____

    No _____

Comments: _____

_____

_____

16. Rate your overall performance as a member of this board.

Unsatisfactory 1 -- 2 -- 3 -- 4 -- 5 -- 6 -- 7 -- 8 -- 9 -- 10 Satisfactory

Source: Witt Associates Inc.

Board-rating evaluation. Finally, the board-rating method is one in which board members rate one another's performance in a variety of areas. This allows directors to take a thorough look at total board performance. Some topics, such as rating the board chairperson, are untouchable issues in certain boardrooms, while other boards seek out comments on the style of the chairperson and committee chairpersons. The results are presented confidentially to these people on an individual basis.

One board I worked with had an attorney who was written into the bylaws by name as the chairperson of the board and as chairperson of the executive, finance, and nominating committees. Other board members, predictably, understood their roles to be subservient. When the ratings of his performance were less than he would have preferred, this chairperson simply omitted the discussion of that issue.

For a board to profit from any form of evaluation, it may need a full day's meeting to process the results. Discussions should always result in a "to-do" list for the board.

Failure to correct, change, and improve board performance will lower morale. The better board members will leave if they sense a lack of opportunity to learn and grow. Or, rather than leaving, board members may simply put in their time and create an appropriate reason for not standing for reelection at the end of their term.

Fortunately, hospital boards today are awakening to the need to improve their own performance. They are becoming much more active in pursuing opportunities to learn about their responsibilities and performance.

The following sample evaluation could be used to help board members rate total board performance.

Sample Board-Rating Evaluation

This questionnaire asks you to evaluate your hospital board. All ratings will be collected and tabulated and the results will be presented for discussion.

Person completing is a member of:

Board _____   Management _____   Medical Staff _____

1. The board periodically reviews the mission statement and corporate objectives to determine both current and future direction of the institution.

   Never 1---- 2---- 3---- 4---- 5---- 6---- 7---- 8---- 9---- 10 Always

2. The board understands and accepts its responsibility for reviewing the appropriateness of long-range planning and corporate strategy.

   Never 1---- 2---- 3---- 4---- 5---- 6---- 7---- 8---- 9---- 10 Always

3. The board assists management to review its short- and long-range planning assumptions as they relate to economic, political, and market projections.

   Never 1---- 2---- 3---- 4---- 5---- 6---- 7---- 8---- 9---- 10 Always

4. The board periodically studies the institution's competitive position in its market by assisting management to review comparative trends and data concerning similar organizations.

   Never 1---- 2---- 3---- 4---- 5---- 6---- 7---- 8---- 9---- 10 Always

5. Does the management information system for the organization allow for sophisticated planning techniques?

   No _____   Yes _____

6. Does the board regularly refer to approved goals, objectives, and plans to guide its decision-making process?

   No _____   Yes _____

7. Is there an understanding and acceptance that the organization is managed and led by the CEO, who serves at the pleasure of the board?

   No _____ Yes _____

8. Does the board understand its need for a succession plan for the position of CEO that includes how people will be identified, reviewed, and selected—whether internally or externally?

   No _____ Yes _____

9. Does the board have a succession plan for itself, in terms of how board members are identified, reviewed, and selected?

   No _____ Yes _____

10. Does the board have a written conflict of interest policy that reviews annually any board member's business that does business with the hospital?

    No _____ Yes _____

11. Other than their board service, are there any services that are sold to the institution by members of the board?

    None   1----2----3----4----5----6----7----8----9----10   Many

12. Has the board's structure been designed to help the institution achieve its purposes and goals?

    No _____ Yes _____

13. Does the board have an adequate range of expertise and board experience to make it effective?

    No _____ Yes _____

14. Are the majority of directors devoting adequate time to their board responsibilities?

    No _____ Yes _____

15. Should the board consider changes in its bylaws concerning any of the following:

    Board size?

    No _____ Yes _____

    Age composition?

    No _____ Yes _____

    Sex composition?

    No _____ Yes _____

Geographical composition?

No _____   Yes _____

Tenure in office?

No _____   Yes _____

Compensation?

No _____   Yes _____

Membership on boards or partnerships of competing organizations?

No _____   Yes _____

16. Should the committee system be reviewed and revised?

No _____   Yes _____

17. Do all committees have written statements of purpose?

No _____   Yes _____

18. Do all board members serve on at least one committee?

No _____   Yes _____

19. How would you rate the chairperson's ability to run effective meetings?

Low 1-----2-----3-----4-----5-----6-----7-----8-----9-----10 High

20. Does the chairperson of the board have a written position description and personal specifications?

No _____   Yes _____

21. How would you rate the board's ability to focus on substantial policy matters as opposed to minutiae and administrative details?

Low 1-----2-----3-----4-----5-----6-----7-----8-----9-----10 High

22. Does a specific committee (i.e., executive compensation, audit, or personnel) have responsibility for evaluation of the CEO's performance and compensation?

No _____   Yes _____

23. Does the board have a list of specifications for board membership?

No _____   Yes _____

24. Does the board do a strengths and weaknesses audit to pinpoint areas of expertise that it lacks?

No _____   Yes _____

25. Does the board have a disciplinary policy for board members?

    No _____   Yes _____

26. Does it have a plan to get rid of non-contributing board members?

    No _____   Yes _____

27. Does the board understand and accept its fiduciary accountability in areas of financial performance?

    No _____   Yes _____

28. Does the board regularly get financial information and data that are understandable, timely, and useful?

    No _____   Yes _____

29. Does the board feel there is adequate opportunity to discuss trends in the organization's financial performance?

    No _____   Yes _____

30. Does the board have an approved audit policy, and does it review the implementation of auditor recommendations?

    No _____   Yes _____

31. Does the board annually approve and select outside auditors?

    No _____   Yes _____

32. Does the board have a written policy and procedure for CEO evaluation and compensation?

    No _____   Yes _____

33. Does the board have an established set of performance standards or criteria that allow for periodic evaluation of a director's performance?

    No _____   Yes _____

34. Does the board understand the art of asking penetrating, pertinent questions?

    No _____   Yes _____

35. Does the board have an educational development policy with annual time requirements for all directors?

    No _____   Yes _____

36. Does the CEO have the necessary authority to manage the corporation?

    No _____   Yes _____

37. Does the board understand the need to ensure that the institution is understood and appreciated by its publics?

    No _____   Yes _____

38. Do board members share market information or perspectives from their outside worlds with the organization's CEO?

    No _____   Yes _____

39. Do board members occasionally request additional financial information for their own edification or clarification?

    No _____   Yes _____

40. How would you rate the credibility and trust between the board and the CEO?

    Low 1-----2-----3-----4-----5-----6-----7-----8-----9-----10 High

41. How would you rate the advance information materials you receive for board meetings?

    Low 1-----2-----3-----4-----5-----6-----7-----8-----9-----10 High

Source: Witt Associates Inc.

Processing the Results

When answering questions about one's own board performance or about the total board, the benefits will double if the results are distributed and discussed. Reviewing results has proven to be an excellent springboard to discussion in every seminar I've ever done. Obviously we're not talking about someone else, now—this is very personal. Most boards will repeat the experience once they have completed it.

For example, in the self-rating method, members examine the summary report of how members rated themselves and how they compare their own score to a composite score of the group on each question. In the board-rating method, individuals rate the board as a whole on a variety of factors or questions and look for areas of weakness or questions that require discussion. In yet another approach, the board's self-evaluation can be compared to the CEO's evaluation of the board, and then discussed. The latter becomes appropriate when a board accepts the fact that the CEO as an agent of the board is an integral part of board effectiveness.

Such a discussion at a two-day board retreat can lead to a long list of changes the board will want to implement to improve its performance and effectiveness.

Any board willing to pursue the evaluation exercise with a seeking, searching attitude will be rewarded. Board evaluation results in board development, which repays all involved.

7.

The Board Chairperson's Responsibilities

The position of board chairperson suffers in most hospitals from a total lack of definition. People assume the chairperson will "run the board meetings" or "direct the board." In fact, most chairs handle the job by recalling their own experience on other boards or that of role models on the hospital board.

In many public corporations, the CEO assumes the additional role of chairperson. In those cases, the CEO usually has years of service and knows the organization intimately. Investing all that power and authority in one person ensures a strong, effective course for the enterprise. In such situations, the board is there to advise and counsel a knowledgeable leader. It does not see its role as controlling or directing an amateur or a hired hand.

All this is not true for hospital board chairpersons. Board members have little or no training in institutional management with its multidisciplinary environment. A volunteer board chairperson usually serves one or two years and rotates. Without a position description to guide new persons, performance becomes inconsistent.

In the past 20 years, hospital boards have moved away from the self-perpetuating model in which the only limitation to a person's board term was death itself. Self-perpetuation usually made for boards loaded with conservative, analytical men and women who did not serve as *rudders* to the institution, but as *anchors*. Then the Joint Commission on the Accreditation of Hospitals partially solved this problem by pushing for specified terms for board members. But I think we threw some babies out with that bathwater.

Experience shows that in both non-profit and for-profit enterprises the best results have been achieved by long-term service from both a board chairperson and a CEO. In top American companies, those two key spots are stable positions. The best community hospitals have always had stability in those two leadership roles. A good working relationship of long standing between the CEO and board chairperson is the best combination for organizational success.

A hospital board will not play an effective role in the organization unless it is capable of managing its own affairs. This means that a person who leads and manages the board must be selected to do a well-defined job. Failure to define this position leaves the board open to "some good years" and "some bad years." A board that treats the chairperson's position too casually need not look very far if it is unsatisfied with the organization's progress.

I'd like to comment on each aspect of a sample position description for a hospital board chairperson. Perhaps this will provide food for thought during the next discussions of the board's nomination committee.

Sample Position Description
for Board Chairperson

Basic Function

The chairperson shall manage the affairs of the board of directors.

Specific Duties

1. The chairperson shall preside over all meetings of the board of directors and the executive committee.
2. The chairperson shall oversee all committees to ensure that they are efficient and productive.
3. The chairperson is responsible for periodic assessment of the individual directors, discipline of board members, the committees of the board, and the board as a whole.
4. The chairperson is responsible for recruitment, orientation, and development of all board members.
5. The chairperson is responsible for board agendas and preparation of the advance information packet.
6. The chairperson is responsible for directing the internal audit.
7. The chairperson is responsible for maintenance of the policy manual and the board manual.

Personal Qualifications

1. Board experience in corporations of equivalent size to the hospital.
2. Extensive experience in development of corporate strategies for successful organizations.

3. Experience in multidimensional or high-technology business.
4. Experience in disciplines such as corporate negotiations, marketing, and new product or service development.

Source: Witt Associates Inc.

Responsibilities of the Board Chairperson

After reviewing literally thousands of hospital bylaws it's possible for me to state that they simply do not define a chairperson's responsibility. The most common boilerplate language sounds about like this one from a Cleveland Hospital.

The chairman shall preside at all meetings of the Board, and shall be, ex officio, a member of all committees. The chairman shall have such other powers and duties as incumbent upon the chairman of a voluntary non-profit corporation or as are imposed by law, or as may from time to time be assigned by the Board.

The responsibilities of the board chairperson involve fundamental duties. Each board may decide on slightly different responsibilities but these are basic to almost any situation:

Preside over board meetings. This sounds easy, but few people conduct meetings properly. A good chair knows when to limit discussion. For example, if the board falls into the trap of rehashing what was decided in committee, it's the board chairperson's responsibility to get things back on track. Tact and diplomacy are needed. Some chairpersons dominate meetings excessively while others exercise so little direction that board meetings become a source of aggravation.

Meetings should be run efficiently and the key player in this process is the chair. Actually, every two or three years, a worthwhile topic for a board development session is meeting dynamics or how to improve meeting results.

Oversee all committees. Generally, the chairperson is responsible for the organization of committees and task forces.

This includes clarifying the purpose of each committee, and assigning the proper persons to each committee to create the best mix of talents and interests.

In the best-organized boards, chairperson supervision of committees may also include monitoring standards of performance and annually evaluating committee work. Ineffective committees should have their purposes revised, renewed, or the mix of members changed.

In some organizations, the chairperson is at least an ex officio member of all committees. How the total board and its committees function is the responsibility of the chairperson. When any part of the board mechanism does not operate effectively, the chair should be held accountable.

Assess individual director performance and group effectiveness. While some boards view this as a one-time exercise, truly effective organizations will make this an annual event. One reason evaluation of boards is rarely done is that responsibility for the task is never assigned. I would suggest you make the chair responsible for this assessment process.

Whether the chairperson uses a board committee or an outside consultant is unimportant. The major result should be that any necessary changes or corrections are implemented as quickly as possible. If the chair has this responsibility, there is little excuse for lack of remedial action or follow-up.

Discipline of volunteers sounds inappropriate but it is very necessary. The chairperson must be responsible for the board member who starts individual negotiations with outside parties with no direction or approval from the board, the board member who leaks confidential information consistently, and the non-performing member who doesn't attend 50 percent of the meetings. The chair must control the proverbial "loose cannon on the deck."

Recruit, orient, and develop board members. This is another process that is handled far too casually in most organizations. The process of finding and selecting new board members is absolutely essential to corporate survival, but it is too often viewed as a once-a-year activity. In fact, it should be a persistent concern for the board chairperson. The wise chairperson will do an annual audit of the background experience of each of the directors. When a void is uncovered or anticipated, finding a person with the right experience or contacts will become a priority. The chair should be held accountable for the quality of the people on the board.

The sensitive chairperson will seek to identify training and development needs for individual directors and for the total board. Commonly, the board retreat program is planned by the CEO, and the board chairperson is an interested spectator. I believe he or she needs to be involved fully in the process, charged with the responsibility for board development.

Prepare agenda and advance-information packages. While in most hospitals the CEO prepares board agendas in cooperation with the board chairperson, the ultimate accountability attaches to the chair. The board meeting will be run by the chairperson and he or she should have control of the agenda. Review of all information, proposals, plans, and strategies to be presented to the full board is a natural responsibility. A working chairperson will poll members in advance on agenda items to make sure that all information that may be requested can be gathered in time. This provides a meeting with few surprises and leaves almost no items placed on the table for another month or two while facts and figures are collected for presentation.

Most board members are not associated with the health care business in any substantial way. Thus, the board must receive an adequate supply of information prior to board and committee meetings to properly serve the corporation and support management. Some of those information needs will be about the hospital in general, about the industry, background information for agenda items, feedback on operations, or progress of members of management.

Maintain policy and board manuals. These documents guide and facilitate the board's activities. They catalog policies, procedures, and current position descriptions for the board, its officers, the CEO, and all committees. They include policy statements adopted by the board, grouped in logical sequence. Any board member can use them to understand the character, culture, values, needs, and stages of growth through which the corporation has evolved. The responsibility for these manuals rests with the chairperson.

Personal Characteristics

The person who chairs a board needs certain personal qualities to execute the position's responsibilities efficiently. Positions of power, influence, and responsibility require people with integrity, courage, commitment, independence, good faith, good will, and strength enough to admit when they need help. While it may sound like the Scout oath to some, these factors should nevertheless be used to judge candidates for the chair position.

Integrity. If the person in the chair is anything less than honest, both board and CEO will waste a lot of time and energy. In every dealing, both internal and external, the chairperson must be aware that he or she is establishing the corporate value system. That value system must reflect integrity and honorable purposes. Wheelers and dealers as board chairpersons can turn a hospital boardroom into a political arena.

Courage. The duties of a board chairperson frequently call for the ability to resist pressures and to be fair, consistent, and objective. Objectivity in particular is not easy. However, the courageous chair will hear all the alternatives in any discussion. If the situation demands, a chairperson may step down during a particular discussion and let someone else chair the meeting.

Board chairpersons, in my experience, have been heavily pressured from time to time by medical staffs, regulatory agencies, competitive hospitals, employee groups, and fellow board members. How they handle that pressure is critical. I remember a bank president who served as board chairperson of a hospital. The hospital's strategic plan called for primary care clinics in outreach areas, but the doctors lobbied the chairperson with threats that they would seek another bank if the board did not stop being "disloyal" to its medical staff. He did not knuckle under, and the threats were not carried out.

Commitment. The key issue is: Who will stand up for the institution and its mission? Let me illustrate this as I do in board retreats: A new hospital board chairperson announces that his motivation for serving on the board is to reduce health care costs. It sounds downright noble! But that chairperson has a personal agenda—cutting costs—that will affect all of his decisions about hospital policy. Whenever the board discusses issues that involve money, this new chairperson's primary consideration will not be what is best for the hospital, but what will cut hospital costs. The board chairperson needs to be committed first and foremost to the hospital and its mission. All other loyalties must be secondary to this main commitment.

Independence. There are different kinds of independence, and all of them are desirable. If the chairperson is financially independent, he or she can afford to be courageous and objective. Independence also means an individual does not need to take the job for real or imagined gains. The best board chairpersons I've seen have had a large amount of independence with a generous amount of humility and compassion.

The chair must be able to participate in major decisions and in the development of corporate policies free from outside influence. Allowing a fair hearing to all sides despite lobbying efforts is not easy, but it is the chairperson's responsibility.

Good faith/good will. With competitive pressures and the many controversial issues that arise from patient complaints, medical staff quality problems, and biomedical ethics questions, the person who does not possess an innate good faith and a belief in people's unlimited capacity for good will find the board chairperson position an unbearable hot seat.

Willingness to ask for help. The modern health care organization can confront people with situations and circumstances they have never faced before. The ability to admit ignorance and to get the necessary help is a great strength. The biggest problems I've seen at the board level occurred when the board tried to decide a tough issue without help. No one has ever built a monument to a *thrifty* board or CEO, and yet many boards feel that they are saving money by not getting the best advice available. Some board chairpersons feel it is a badge of honor not to pay for help when evaluating their CEO. One hospital I know has lost two good CEOs in the last six years, and the third is looking for another job. But they continue to think they know enough not to need help.

Experience. The candidate for chairperson of a hospital board should possess a blend of skills and experience. These might include board experience, management experience, marketing experience with consumer products and services, and strategic planning experience.

The board chairperson needs to "fit" in the same way that the CEO does. I've seen a board chairperson for a $20 million hospital organization who personally never worked in an organization with more than 15 employees and $1 million in gross sales. Yet, I know that if a candidate from a 40-bed hospital were presented for a CEO position in that 200-bed hospital, the board would laugh the candidate right out of consideration.

To help strengthen boards overnight, I suggest requiring that the chairperson have hospital board experience of at least five years. This would add depth and perspective to the chairperson's position, certainly. Everyone agrees that hospitals are complex, competitive businesses, so it is time to recognize the key role of the board chairperson.

Managing the affairs of the board and leading the board in its supervision of the total operation requires a real appreciation for both the theory and practice of management. A chair needs to understand what a CEO faces in the job. It's no accident that the most common occupation of board members in public corporations is active or retired CEO. People who have been in the position can appreciate what it takes to implement the board's objectives.

Experience in organizations that had to adjust to changing markets is invaluable. Hospitals are driven partially by high technology and partially by competing forces. Add to this the government's constant changing of the rules, and it becomes apparent that almost any course of action must be subject to change. Frequently board members complain about crisis management and last-minute decisions. This is simply a reflection of the environment in which all hospitals are continually fighting for position.

The chairperson's position was for years a sought-after title that carried prestige, power, and influence—but in many places it became a perfunctory role. Now the times are changing, and the position is no longer honorary or ceremonial. Instead, the chairperson is a vital member of the hospital team.

A few institutions have recognized the growing role of the chairperson. They have named their long-term CEO to the chairperson role. These people have obviously built up years of personal and professional credibility. It's an idea whose time may be coming. Every board should at least discuss the concept. The results of such discussion may give a good indication of how businesslike they really wish to become.

Corporate strategy. Unless a person has had experience in the development and implementation of corporate plans, this can be a problem area. Sound corporate strategy is not developed by committees. Strategy is developed by staff, then shaped and molded by board discussion. Persons not familiar with corporate planning processes will perhaps have a longer learning curve. They also may not understand the lead times necessary in strategic planning. The more board experience in corporate planning the board chairperson and other board members have, the better able they are to assess management's recommendations in this key area.

Multidisciplinary environments. If a board chairperson

comes from a fairly well-defined business such as banking, retailing, or manufacturing, everything seems black and white. The hospital organization is a complex organization with political and professional ties that will confuse many business leaders. It's almost like the businessman who was appointed to a high government position in Washington. After his first year, he was asked what the job was like and he replied, "It's like pushing on a wall made of jelly. As soon as you remove your hand, it goes back to its original shape."

For people who lack the perspective, the hospital organization can be a real maze. Candidates for chairperson need as much exposure to complex but successful organizations as they can get.

Negotiations, marketing, or product development. Board chairpersons with business experience in one of these three key areas can be a real plus. As hospitals seek to prosper in what appears to be a hostile environment, certain experience can be invaluable. If the environment changes, persons with productivity or financial functional experience may be needed. The point is that both the board and management will be helped by a board chairperson with strong functional skills.

Achievement. It seldom gets talked about, but it needs to be mentioned. Because the board chairperson's job has both status and power, it can be dangerous if awarded to the wrong person. Try to select someone who has achieved in his or her own career. People who accept the position as having more power and status than anything they've ever experienced may lose their heads in the excitement and make some foolish mistakes.

Most corporations of any size have a person who achieved personal and professional success long before becoming a board chairperson. That individual has the perspective and has paid the price. He or she has had the opportunity to experience pressures from below, above, and externally. All this is excellent training.

A middle manager of a major corporation who had been in

a staff role for his entire career was the most dangerous board chairperson I've ever seen. He was out to prove his corporate employer had made a mistake and that he was really presidential timber. He was so wrong!

A humorous but sad case was the attorney of a two-member law firm who ran the board as a plaything for 10 years. He called meetings at whatever time or place he felt necessary. This resulted in five board meetings one month and none for the next four, and a chaotic governance pattern for the organization.

Neither of these gentlemen should have been a board chairperson. Do *you* have any stories to share on the subject?

8.

Hiring the Chief Executive Officer

The most important responsibility for any hospital board is hiring the best chief executive possible. Successful boards seek to attract someone who can lead them and the organization, a chief executive of vision and courage who will surround himself or herself with a team of other capable executives.

When a vacancy occurs in the chief executive's position, the board simultaneously faces its greatest responsibility and its greatest opportunity. Today's health care business is understood by few board members; a wise board realizes that it needs someone to educate, inform, and lead both the board and the organization.

Vacancies in the CEO position occur in four basic situations, with a multitude of variations. Retirement can occur either early or on a date set by the incumbent. Voluntary separation usually involves the incumbent's departure to accept another position. Forced separation occurs when a board asks a chief executive to leave (regardless of how the separation is camouflaged). Death or disability of the CEO is obviously the least expected cause of a vacancy.

Retirement

Retirement vacancies can occur in a variety of ways. If there is a board policy and a retirement program, the situation is easily handled. I've seen cases where CEOs had no desire to leave although the board felt it was time for a change. Or, I've watched CEOs without adequate retirement income make a board feel guilty enough to keep them past normal retirement age. Then again, some CEOs should be encouraged to take early retirement. These types frequently hold back a whole management team so as not to rock the boat before they retire. An organization can lose momentum in these situations. It's happening every day all across the country.

The biggest problems can occur when an organization with a CEO age 58 or more tries to hire a much younger number two person. Younger people know they'll be judged on how much they can accomplish, which may mean changes. Incumbent CEOs may not view changes to "their organization" very kindly. The games that get played in these situations can be prevented if a board clearly spells out the time lines it is working with, the results it expects, and the terms of the CEO stepping aside, even when that is an early retirement. I'll discuss examples in the chapter on compensation.

Some CEOs will not want their board members to read this—but retirement of the CEO is a board's prerogative. I refer to this as a "bad-breath" topic, because no one wants to talk about the subject. I've also noticed that boards start to think silently about the subject when CEOs reach age 57 or 58, regardless of how good their performance records are to that point. Obviously, when the board members have questions about performance and achievement, they will start to think about retirement even earlier.

The reason this subject is discussed in this chapter is that the way a board handles its current CEO may greatly affect the quality of future candidates for the position. This area requires objectivity, sensitivity, and decisiveness. Boards that try to please all parties may handle the situation poorly.

Voluntary Separation

This can be easy or difficult, depending on how much communication the parties are willing to engage in before the fact. Standards that are discussed usually are taken from a general employee relations norm that says employees should give a termination notice equal to the vacation time they receive. Two weeks' vacation means two weeks' notice, and so on.

For CEOs and boards, the practice is normally two or three months in theory, although less in practice. Once a CEO announces his or her departure, the board and management will begin to make their own decisions or go around the "lame duck." Nevertheless, a few months notice is pretty standard.

The same small committee that reviewed the CEO's performance should conduct an exit interview. The following questions are a small sample of what the board might ask:

1. What did you enjoy most about the position?
2. What did you enjoy least?
3. What are the organization's three major problems (challenges) for your successor?
4. What are the organizations' three major strengths?
5. What are the board's greatest strengths and greatest improvement needs?
6. What are the three biggest competitors to the organization?
7. What are the medical staff's strength and weaknesses?
8. If your brother-in-law or daughter were applying for this position, what would you tell them?

Forced Separation

Forced separation is traumatic. A board needs an effective CEO it can trust, or else it will constantly want to do management's job. When second-guessing and friction become the climate of board meetings, the board should determine whether the majority of the board lack faith in the CEO. If the board has established goals and objectives and it feels the CEO has not accomplished satisfactory results then it is best to part with the CEO. A fair settlement will allow adequate severance for the CEO. The amount is usually related to tenure with the organization and the CEO's age. As these factors increase, so will the severance.

A board that maintains a person as CEO after it is clear that the relationship is not working has become part of the problem. At that point, the board shares a responsibility for the failure. I watched one internally promoted CEO who had spent eight years previously as a vice-president. When his boss died suddenly, he was promoted; and within two years the board knew it had made a mistake. But it wasn't until ten years later that a new board chairperson asked the 51-year-old CEO to leave. Clearly, that organization owed its CEO a generous settlement. More about that in a later chapter.

Death or Disability

Every board should have a "succession discussion" once each year to decide what it would do if the CEO died. Disability is another matter, and it's wise to think about how your board would handle a CEO with a lingering illness.

Any contract or retirement plan should provide for early retirement. This is not a one-way provision for the benefit of the CEO, because it also allows a board to move fairly and decisively when it feels the organization is losing momentum. This is another of those "bad-breath" topics that needs discussion in every board room *before* it is an emergency.

A Change of Leadership

In any event, a change of leadership can be a refreshing experience. A new executive should bring new ideas, methods, and outlooks, and this change should be used to advantage. The need for a new CEO creates an opportunity for the board to reevaluate the organization and reassess its objectives. This is not a casual decision. Occasionally, institutions will panic when they find themselves without a CEO. They will hire the first available candidate or elevate someone internally, only to regret that hasty action later. Even when a strong candidate is available from within, wise boards seek other applicants to give perspective to their final decision. Not just a "whitewash" to make their internal choice look good, the national search will truly give the organization the best person.

When a board appoints an internal candidate without interviewing at least three outside candidates, it misses a rare opportunity to question, analyze, evaluate, and assess different management styles. If the internal person is an excellent candidate, he or she will compare favorably with other candidates. If not, those comparisons could save the board the embarrassment of having to change executives again in the near future. Many a board has regretted an emotional decision that appointed a long-time vice-president who was great as a number two person, but who lacks something as the CEO. My advice to boards that are ready to appoint internally is to call six board members from organizations that two years previously made an internal appointment and listen to what they tell you. A thorough national executive search is the best insurance for the most important decision a board ever makes.

Boards should also be cautious about appointing *acting* chief executives. The internal candidate who has an acting role may perform impartially while awaiting the board's best objective decision, but some acting executives move into the chief executive's office, promote subordinates, grant management pay increases, hire new key personnel, and take other major actions to curry the favor of management, board, and staff.

I've seen instances where an in-house candidate used the professional grapevine to discourage qualified people from considering the position, by putting out the word that he or she was the front runner. Worse yet, I've seen boards that were sure their internal candidate was the world's greatest, having made no comparisons at all.

The internal promotion is a real temptation, but some people are not qualified to move up to number one. They weren't selected with that thought in mind, they weren't given those kinds of responsibilities, and they may not have the personality for it. If you are looking at a vice-president who *might* be qualified to move up, you should always make comparisons with outside candidates, even if you think you have the greatest person in the world. Committees should not select from a universe of one, because that leaves them open forever to the charge that they didn't make a prudent choice.

The main point for board members to remember is that hiring and firing the chief executive is the most basic responsibility they have. If they handle it well, they won't need to do it often. But when they are faced with the task, they should take the time to select the best person. Resisting medical staff politicking for their choice is something few boards are able to do. The same campaigning may take place by elements of the board. The question remains: Is the person to whom we're offering the CEO job the *best* person?

The Selection Committee

A committee is undoubtedly needed for the process of hiring. These committees have been misnamed search committees, when in fact they should be selection committees. An organization that uses a so-called search committee runs the risk that the committee will find a candidate whom the rest of the board will turn down. The board should understand that it is delegating the responsibility to a committee to make a *final* recommendation to the full board. University medical centers are famous for searches that take 12 to 18 months. After all the logrolling and campaigning is over, the person they select may simply be the best politician, not the best candidate. If they get a real leader, it's more by accident than design.

The selection committee is a working committee, rarely composed of more than five members, although some have been effective with seven. A larger committee usually becomes unwieldy and functions slowly and inefficiently. The previous board chairperson, the current chairperson, and the future chairperson are generally an excellent starting group, plus other interested, qualified board members. Non-board members, whether members of management or staff, have no place on the committee. This is the board members' responsibility, and they should carry it out.

The committee chairperson should be appointed for his or her ability to guide and direct group activity. Autocratic leaders make bad chairpersons because their decisions may be subject to second-guessing. The excessively democratic leader is an equally poor choice because, in an eagerness to achieve 100 percent consensus, this leader may delay final decisions unnecessarily.

Just as an effective committee needs authority to act, so must the chairperson possess leadership to get things done in a climate of mutual respect. Many good prospects are lost to procrastination or lack of organization by the selection committee.

I recall all too vividly a hospital selection committee that insisted on having seven board members, five physicians, and two members of management. It took weeks to get a majority of the 14-member committee to schedule the first interview. It took over two months to complete three candidate interviews! Then the candidates were kept waiting six weeks while the committee decided who should be the final two to invite back for second visits. To shorten a long, tragic story, they were turned down by a candidate who had waited six months from his first visit. The committee never could get past a seven-to-seven vote. So much for democracy and consensus!

The selection committee should represent many viewpoints among the board of directors. For instance, there may be directors who feel that the CEO should concentrate on medical staff relations. Other directors may believe the greatest problems are financial; hence, the executive they prefer would be well-versed in financial management. Some will prefer a young candidate, while others seek maturity. Some may feel marketing will be the greatest challenge to the organization, while others feel that quality of care will sell the institution.

Whenever possible, include board members on this committee who have had some prior involvement with executive selection in their own business. People who have operated a one-person shop or family business may lack the perspective necessary for selecting a chief executive who will inherit a large workforce and complexities unknown to the small-business person. Such people tend to select executives whom they'd like to have as friends, who would be companionable guests for dinner. The small operator may find it awkward to think in terms of a job that carries a starting salary greater than his or her own income.

The selection committee needs representatives from various groups, interests, and positions. If the organization has had any political turmoil, see to it that the various factions on the board are represented. Make certain that people who have differing opinions or philosophies about the kind and type of organization they ought to have, and about what kind of person ought to run it, are on the committee. The charge to the committee should be quite specific: "To find, attract, select, and recommend to the full board for its approval a candidate for the key executive position."

Hiring a Search Consultant

The search process today requires time, expertise, and energy. A group of volunteers on a committee is simply not equipped to find somebody to run their business. Writing letters and asking people for names is amateurish and can lead to real problems. To be objective, thorough, and responsible in this process, the board should retain an executive search consultant. This may sound self-serving, but it is the truth. The organization needs somebody who can give it the time, energy, and education that it will almost surely require throughout a successful search assignment.

A lot of cumbersome detail work goes into finding and selecting a new CEO. The committee should seek consulting assistance from an organization that knows the health field. Health care is a uniquely specialized business, and general executive search experience won't help a consultant who doesn't understand how voluntary boards operate. It is seldom necessary to interview more than three consultants. You can get names of search consulting firms from these three sources:

— American Association of Hospital Consultants, Arlington, Virginia. (Some of their members do executive search work.)

— Association of Executive Search Consultants, Greenwich, Connecticut. (Some of their members are qualified to do health care searches.)

— Chairpersons of search committees at other organizations that filled a position in the last two or three years. (Their personal experience should be helpful.)

Working with a Search Consultant

The first step for a search consultant is to define with you both the job your organization wants done and the characteristics of persons likely to be acceptable to your selection committee. Most selection committee members feel that this process is unnecessary until they are asked the question, "What three things would you like to see the CEO complete in the first year on the job that would cause you to give the highest pay raise you've ever given?" It gets very, very quiet as the committee members try to express specifically what they are looking for.

Many of the same problems occur as committee members define the experience and style they want in candidates. Because a person has a degree in health care administration, or has worked as a vice-president, chief operating officer, or chief executive, it does not necessarily follow that the person is compatible with your institution.

Very different skills stand out in the chief executive of a small community institution when compared to the executive of a major teaching hospital. The CEO of a smaller facility may be extremely familiar with capital financing, staffing issues, quality assurance, or politics, while a candidate from a multifacility organization may be in a better position to see the broad issues in health care, have a stronger corporate orientation, and better understand joint ventures from actual experience. Some organizations can profit from employing a young, creative, energetic go-getter, while a more traditional board could be stumbling into an untenable situation by hiring the proverbial "young tiger."

The executive search consultant helps the organization to understand its own needs, both immediate and long-term. Sometimes, an organization has had a great deal of turmoil and stress—a real struggle with a competing hospital, a merger that failed, a scandal within the hospital, a fight among the medical staff. The most immediate need is for a knight in shining armor. They want credibility—somebody who is married, with 2.5 kids, who salutes the flag every morning, pays his taxes early, and leads the Fourth of July parade. Such people exist but they're not easy to find. Most boards have ideal specifications for a candidate but will settle for something less than perfection.

If a board actually finds the "perfect" CEO (whatever that means to them), it must be remembered that such people want to be treated very differently than does the average person. The outstanding individual will require special handling.

When an organization has been standing still for years, board members may think they need somebody to come in, take some actions, make some decisions, and move things in a hurry. The committee has to recognize that its unique circumstances will require a certain type of person.

Statement of Purpose

Earlier in the book, I suggested that each board committee should have a statement of purpose and job description. Here is a sample of one for the selection committee.

Sample Selection Committee Statement of Purpose and Job Description

Reports to: Board of Directors

Statement of Purpose

To find, attract, select, and recommend to the full board for its approval a candidate for the chief executive position.

Duties

— Assess the organization's strengths and weaknesses.

— Interview three executive search consultants, check at least four references on each one, and select a consultant to do the staff work.

— Establish job and personal specifications for the position with consultant assistance.

— Establish a reasonable schedule for finding, screening, and investigating potential candidates.

— Report on progress at least monthly to the full board.

— Meet as necessary and communicate regularly with the search consultant to provide necessary information and data for candidates.

— Meet with the search consultant to decide on the final three or four candidates to be interviewed.

— Serve as hosts to candidates and their spouses during the interview process.

— Interview, individually or as a group, all candidates during a hospital visit.

— Be ready (chairperson and one other member) to travel to meet with candidates, if necessary.

— Ensure that references on the final candidate have been checked by the consultant.

— Coordinate any personal reference checks with the chairperson of the committee and the consultant to prevent candidate embarrassment and preserve hospital good will.

— Formally evaluate the final acceptable candidates and decide who the candidate of choice will be. (Chairperson will negotiate, with consultant assistance, with the final candidate.)

— Release suitable public announcements of the appointment both internally and externally.

Source: Witt Associates Inc.

Making Decisions

Many boards will defend their right to make certain decisions but will suddenly waffle on this one and become accommodating to everyone—the medical staff, ladies' auxiliary, or town council. If you ask the board whether it is running a social service or a business, it would be quick to respond that, with a $10 million or $50 million or $100 million budget, the hospital is a business. But many board members still perceive the hospital as more of a social service agency than a business. They suddenly become more interested in pleasing imagined constituencies than in achieving organization results, goals, and objectives.

The businesslike way to go about the selection process is to be objective and firm, to have a definite idea in mind of what you want, and then go for it. But hospital boards will often try to reach a consensus. Most business boards are not required to pick somebody who is politically acceptable to customers, employees, and business associates. Chrysler Corp. would have made an absolute fool of itself if it had asked the workers, the dealers, and suppliers to vote on Iaccoca. Can you guess the answer if they had gone out to the dealers and asked whether they would like to have a former Ford executive as the Chrysler CEO? In fact, the Chrysler board went ahead and struck a deal with Iaccoca, and the rest is history—profitable history.

There is no question that selection committee members want to be able to share the risk involved in choosing a CEO; but since this area is at the heart of the board's responsibilities, it has to be objective, willing to take a risk, and willing to hire somebody who is smart, aggressive, a leader.

Boards must guard against making their selection so politically acceptable that they end up with a politician instead of a leader/manager. Few selection committees are honest enough with themselves to accept this as a problem. For example, committees will say they want "a bright, aggressive leader." But candidates who are too outspoken or who demand authority and privileges are, predictably, shot down. When those candidates leave the interview room the committee then complains, "How dare he come in here?" or, "She doesn't know enough about this organization to make those statements!"

On the other hand, few candidates will make firm statements; most will try to be agreeable with the board. What happened to "strong, bright, aggressive"? Gone, gone, gone. Sometimes strong people get by because they apply some of their survival instincts in the interview. They adapt and appear less threatening. And not just in health care—in any field, if people want a job badly enough, they can present themselves in the way they think will be acceptable.

A Word about Number Two People

Heirs apparent in this industry were once established by the chief executives, and usually without a formal vote of a board. Today, though, few health care organizations accept a vice-president as successor to the retiring CEO. CEOs are sometimes guilty of leading on the number two person for years, saying: "When I retire, I'm going to recommend you," but the CEO is the board's choice and those statements are not binding on any board.

The board should know what the chief executive is telling the number two person. Has he or she ever been promised the job? On what basis—tenure and seniority or loyalty? It may not do much damage at lower-level positions to reward loyalty, but it can cause real problems at the chief executive level. What accomplishments and results have these people achieved on their own? Have they been able to disagree with the CEO and push their own ideas and solutions, and have they been successful? Do these people inspire confidence in other managers or are they quietly tolerated?

If it appears I'm too hard on internal candidates it's because few CEOs I know willingly hire strong number two people. In addition, few number two people get both responsibility and authority to function with the board. Finally, few vice-presidents I've known are willing to be objective and change their views when they move up. Yesterday's plans and programs are just fine, thank you.

A new broom will not only sweep clean, but a new executive will not be married to the mistakes of the past. The board will have a rare opportunity to give the organization a shot in the arm by going outside for its top leadership.

The Interview

An interview is an exchange of information. It is also an opportunity to make friends for the institution, and every candidate should be extended the courteous reception accorded to a guest.

The ideal procedure allows the candidate (the invited guest) to be met by a member of the search committee. The two of them can enjoy an informal lunch or dinner while talking as much about the community as the job. This general conversation permits you to get to know the candidate as a person prior to the formal interview.

Following the initial meeting, the committee member should give the visitor a tour of the hospital premises, pointing out those things the facility is most proud of and also problem areas. Occasionally, this tour is conducted by a member of management.

Interviews with key management personnel or key physicians are always of interest to candidates. Their purpose is to give the candidate an opportunity to better understand the organization. But boards convey entirely the wrong message when they ask subordinates to *evaluate* a potential superior.

After the candidate has visited the facility and met various key personnel, an interview with the entire committee is appropriate. The interview becomes much more meaningful for both parties when the candidate is able to relate to the actual physical plant. While the interview should be pleasant and cordial, opening with social amenities, it is nonetheless a meeting with a purpose and should be conducted in a businesslike atmosphere.

Most candidates are not adequately or appropriately interviewed by search committees. The discussion that takes place is little more than polite conversation. In reply to the question, "How did you get along with the staff?" a candidate may say, "I've always gotten along with staff just fine." Although this tells them nothing, some committees will move to another subject. To avoid this kind of unproductive interview technique, the committee should press for examples. What was the candidate's relationship with the board? Ask for specific examples of the person's efforts to educate the board. It is not enough to hold monthly meetings and pass out financial statements and routine reports. Can the applicant cite specific attempts to increase board members' knowledge of a particular area or their understanding of the industry in general? Was the board offered new programs or prepared to meet new trends? These questions should yield details delineating the candidate's contribution to the facility.

I recall one candidate, when asked for his first impression of the institution, who mentioned that he had never seen a sloppier cafeteria. The committee was shaken and, realizing there was an embarrassing element of truth to his observation, shifted gears quickly to another topic. The search committee failed to ask direct questions and gain insight. They could have responded, "Let's assume you are our new chief executive. What would you do in the first 60 to 90 days to improve the food service in our cafeteria and kitchen, and correct the conditions you find so deplorable?" The answers are much more revealing than the questions, but it takes intelligent questioning to produce meaningful answers.

The questions the committee asks should be thought out in advance. A review of the candidate's resumé will raise several logical questions about the candidate's background, experience, and accomplishments. If an applicant mentions, for example, that he or she was successful in restructuring a hospital and personally started six new subsidiary corporations, the committee should probe and inquire about the person's precise role in this process. Did he select the number and type of corporations that were set up? Did she select the managers for each? What were the gross expenses for restructuring? How long did it take all the restructured subsidiaries to pay for the total direct and indirect expenses? How many today are successful businesses, operating at a profit, and showing future growth prospects?

At the end of the interview, the selection committee should determine whether the person would be interested in receiving an offer for the position, and then, when he or she would be available to start working on the new job.

As a courtesy, the committee should conclude each interview by telling the candidates exactly when they can expect a decision, and whether they are still in contention or have been eliminated.

The Selection Process

Isolating the one candidate to whom an offer will be made is the committee's goal. Emotional issues, such as accents or dialects indicative of other regions, golf ability (or its lack), or the fact that the candidate's spouse was born in your state, should play no part in narrowing the selection. The person with the best qualifications overall must surmount the personal interests and prejudices of individual board members.

The selection process is revealing because of the prejudices that surface. Early in the game, when the position's requirements are thrashed out by the selection committee, no hint of personal prejudice usually emerges. In fact, any preferences with regard to age, marital status, or other factors are usually downplayed. Board members are determined to show how liberal and broad-minded they are. But by the time the final selection must be made, all sorts of hitherto unstated conditions have become crucial.

Sometimes, the board selects a candidate who appears to be the type of person they can dominate. The rationale is that this candidate will be easy to live with. Translation: This person won't rock the boat. Is that what the job specifications described? Or did the board say it was looking for a leader, an initiator of programs? Remember, a person who can be dominated by the board may also be dominated by everyone else—staff, community groups, or special interests.

To help the committee make the right decision, each member should have a list of job specifications on hand as each candidate is interviewed. The candidate should be rated on every factor that has been determined to be important—for example, financial management knowledge, decision-making ability, leadership talent, or community affairs.

Many years ago I started using a system to help committees reach an objective choice. A simple numerical point-rating system can be used to compare the candidates. That way, it is possible to see each one's strengths and weaknesses at a glance. Rating is objective and provides a fair assessment of each candidate's fitness for the position. Every candidate is rated on each factor in the specification and points are assigned. An average score is calculated based on everyone's input.

This process should lead the committee to an objective candidate ranking. The position can be offered to the candidate with the best score; if that person turns it down, the committee can move on to candidate number two.

Compensation Considerations

Any candidate who is openly seeking a change will be willing to accept an average salary or only a modest increase for the right opportunity. On the other hand, someone who is being sought, but who is not really dissatisfied enough to be shopping around, will need an improvement over present salary to lure him or her away. A 25 to 30 percent increase in compensation would be a ballpark figure. No one should be offered less than current earnings, nor should people be expected to make a change for essentially the same amount they would receive in another year in their current position. Considering the inherent risk of giving up a sure thing for something unknown, there should be some monetary incentive to motivate the new executive. More on this in chapter 10.

Making the Offer

An offer to the selected candidate should be complete and final. The board has made its decision; the candidate should be expected to make his or hers. No open-ended deals should be offered. Three to seven days should be sufficient time for the candidate to respond to the offer. An exception might be a request for a delay if the candidate wishes to make a family visit to the new locale before committing.

The offer clearly defines starting salary, the type and extent of fringe benefits, and the reporting date. Nothing should be left to chance or worked out after the new executive actually reports. Some details may have to be tailored to fit the candidate, depending on circumstances, but never leave details unresolved.

To present the offer, the chairperson of the selection committee, with whom the candidate is probably best acquainted, should telephone the candidate. Any questions and concerns, such as moving allowances, temporary residences, and the like, can be settled at that time.

Following the phone conversation, the entire offer with all specifics should be confirmed by letter. Request a written acceptance at that time. As long as the candidate seems willing to accept the offer under the terms and conditions prescribed, no further action by the selection committee is required. Only when something of major importance arises, such as a complication with the starting date, should the executive's acceptance be referred to the committee for supplemental approval.

The Closing

It is essential to tell the person you want that you *need* him or her. Say: "We need you because we need the kind of credibility that your personality is going to bring to this organization." Talk about three or four other things and then come back and say again: "We need you in our organization because your ideas and your enthusiasm and energy could really move this hospital." And then you keep talking about some other things and for the third time you come back and say, "You know, we need you," and give another reason why you need them. If those words are spoken in sincerity they are very powerful.

Suppose a candidate has some unresolved questions and you have an articulate, persuasive, and decisive chairperson of your committee. Fly the committee chairperson to the candidate and get things cleared up. That is a great compliment to the candidate and it can effectively close the search.

When the executive has accepted your offer and all the details are arranged, letters of appreciation should go to the other final candidates. At the appropriate time, the organization should distribute a news release announcing the appointment of the new CEO.

Finally, when the new executive and spouse arrive on the scene, they should be given a reception of some sort arranged by the board to let them know they are welcome at the facility and in the community. This gathering should include board members, medical staff, and community leaders. The new executive and family should get started on the right foot, and not feel like outsiders.

That about covers the hiring process for a new chief executive. But the story does not end there; actually, it's only the beginning. Finding the right person for any job is only half the task. The new executive must feel that he or she has found an opportunity that meets or exceeds his or her expectations. In that case, the organization will provide the job satisfaction needed to challenge and satisfy the executive who, in turn, will have that motivation the organization looks for in new leadership.

Other Considerations

The chief executive should have a good team. Good strategic direction for the organization should be evolving through a combination of what management is doing with the board and what the board is doing with management. There should be an atmosphere of growth and development, even if it is a hospital of 50 beds. A 50-bed hospital has a right to grow and get better. It can get cleaner than it was last year, it can be maintained better than it was last year, it can be friendlier, and so on.

Boards tend to focus on either immediate needs or long-term needs. I very seldom see one that can differentiate between the two. If a board feels that it is in a financial crisis, it will look for somebody who is strong in finance, when in fact the right executive can hire a good chief financial officer who can eliminate their financial concerns in a short time. What looks like a financial problem may be a strategic problem. Let a leader decide that.

A hospital board in rural Pennsylvania recently expressed concern about losing their chief executive after only two years on the job. The board couldn't understand how that could happen. I could, once I looked at the individual's previous employment and education. He did not "fit" the situation. A hospital has to make a realistic match to retain an executive for the long term. A small community hospital can *look* at candidates who were raised in large cities and graduated from large universities where they were exposed to all kinds of cultural, social, and entertainment opportunities, but for that type of person to move to a town of 25,000 represents a lifestyle deviation. The candidate may view it as a temporary career move: "I'm going to be here for three years and then I'll be gone." That board should also be willing to look at people who were born and raised in communities of a similar size or who went to school in a smaller community, because small-town life will not require much adjustment. Like the leopard, people just don't change their spots very often.

Hiring the chief executive can be a rewarding learning experience for the board that takes real advantage of the opportunity. After the person is hired, the board's support and encouragement will make it all work. The board that diligently seeks the best CEO it can find, that offers the best package financially, personally, and professionally, and that supports his or her leadership, will have the same feeling that the orchestra musicians feel as they soak up the applause at the end of the evening's performance. Ensemble playing is satisfying.

9.

Evaluating the Chief Executive Officer

It's easy to understand that boards hire and fire the CEO. It's much more difficult to understand why so many boards fail to conduct meaningful performance appraisals of the CEO. Both parties have to communicate in detail about what's wanted, when, and why. Boards of directors must direct the executives they hire. That's what performance appraisal is all about.

If a board (1) understands its cause or mission, and (2) approves the strategies for accomplishing its goals, and (3) *directs* its CEO to achieve those results, the only remaining step is for the board (4) to evaluate the CEO's performance annually. Boards forget that if executives are not clearly guided to what the board wants, they will tend to do what they like to do, or what interests them. Without mutually agreed upon goals it is impossible to pinpoint early problems and to apply corrective measures. And it's amazing how far off the track things can get in a short time.

Even when a direction is established, voluntary boards tend to shift goal emphasis or change priorities, depending on who is on the board. Strong board chairpersons with plenty of time may inappropriately camp on the chief executive's doorstep. They may bury their noses in operations by accident or design. There's real danger here. If the chief executive has allowed the board chairperson to dominate operations, a new chair with a different style can make the board feel that the executive has become ineffective. A new board chairperson and board members may have little time to devote to building a relationship and they may expect the executive to respond quickly to their new style. This is not always possible if there is major turnover on the board every two years. The CEO has to understand and work effectively with these boardroom realities.

It Takes Time

Most boards are looking for a quick way to appraise their CEO's performance. They'll call me and ask for a form or list of factors as if they were doing a performance review of a general office worker. The process deserves more effort because it's much more complex. Each board is different and constantly changing, each organization is different and constantly changing, and every CEO is unique in terms of style and skill. There is no standard form that will fit your individual circumstance.

The reader of this chapter should explore all these elements. Think about the examples and think about your own organization. Evaluating the CEO is a delicate and complex process, which involves superb communication between a board committee and the CEO. It requires openness and candor and, like all relationships, mutual respect.

It is tempting to try and handle this quickly but this is a board responsibility that requires all the time and effort it can get. This is truly board's work. A board committee may get outside, objective advice and counsel, but it alone must take the actions.

The duty of evaluating the CEO is without question the most poorly handled of all board responsibilities. Evaluating the CEO is an art, not a science. It's a process made effective by trial and error. Whatever policies and procedures are established to accomplish evaluation, if communication doesn't take place because of misplaced tact or foolish pride, it's an indictment of that board of directors. This is one time the buck cannot be passed!

To be effective, the process needs to be formalized. Policies, procedures, dates, and time lines need to be set down and agreed on. The process takes time, if it's to be done right, so time must be allocated and spent.

In my board seminars, I often remind board groups that they are governing bodies. They are legally and morally responsible for the corporate organization, its mission, and its people. Of course, the board hires a CEO to manage the organization. A wise and prudent board regularly gets reports from management to assure itself that the corporate mission as well as short- and long-term objectives are being met. The board must oversee management to ensure proper compliance with its own established objectives.

Non-profit hospital organizations have long wrestled with defining what the board does and what management does. As long as boards hesitate to define clearly their own roles, they will be unable to evaluate their CEOs properly. Once a board understands its own responsibilities and spells them out in detail, it is able to define the job of the CEO. Then an annual assessment will be much, much easier for both.

Remember, a group of board members will have different individual ideas about how a CEO and board should function. CEOs can be victims of whisper campaigns that begin harmlessly. One board member asks another: "Does our CEO have the authority to make that kind of decision?" After it's been repeated by another board member or two, the question becomes a statement: "The CEO is headstrong and doesn't consult the board enough."

Without a formal evaluation procedure, many boards historically focus on the CEO's style or personality. One board group in a 400-plus-bed hospital recently gave a new CEO (five months on the job) a letter that questioned his relationships with employees, because he did not eat "often enough" in the employee cafeteria. Another board leaked information to the press on the cost of new furniture for the CEO's office and questioned his judgment. With weak direction and no systematic review of agreed-upon goals and objectives, boards can focus on some very strange things.

Whisper campaigns may begin innocently but they sow the seeds of board discontent, with every board member holding an opinion about what the CEO should be doing and no one entirely satisfied. Unless a formal evaluation policy and procedure are adopted, this second-guessing can continue to perhaps a disastrous conclusion.

The board must approve a policy for an annual evaluation and select a committee to act. When this process is attempted by the full board it becomes a combination kangaroo court and circus.

Policy is the First Step

The best boards see executive evaluation as a regular, annual proposition. They don't wait for a crisis or a confrontation with their chief executive. Instead, they bind themselves to a regular, systematic process to ensure that management is implementing the board's policies. For its part, management is also obligated to report at least annually on performance.

First, the board must agree on its objectives for the evaluation. Some common purposes behind a policy for evaluation are:

— To develop and upgrade the individual skills of the chief executive.

— To reaffirm the strengths of the executive and identify areas for future growth.

— To provide a basis for rewarding the chief executive.

— To allow the board to state its perceptions of executive performance and to allow the executive to agree or disagree.

— To offer proper direction to management on the board's expectations.

Now, some board members look at that list of purposes with a social-service mentality, thinking that the evaluation is an opportunity to correct everything they don't like about their CEO. That's not it. If a behavior doesn't affect performance or the achievement of the organization's goals, it probably isn't appropriate for evaluation. We all have foibles, and some of them just have to be tolerated. Keep an evaluation *businesslike*, at all costs.

Another word of caution: Only the CEO should be the subject of executive evaluation. The board must resist all temptations to evaluate persons who do not report to and are not hired directly by the board. Those evaluations are the responsibility of the individual's immediate superior. Any attempt by the board to influence salary, title, or responsibility of the chief executive's subordinates should be viewed as inappropriate board involvement in operations.

For many years, I have encouraged boards to administer their CEO performance evaluation program with formulated policies that both direct management and guide their board successors. This sample policy from one of our clients could be adapted to fit your individual circumstances.

Sample CEO Evaluation Policy

A performance evaluation shall be conducted annually by a committee of the board. The objectives for the organization that year and any personal objectives for the chief executive officer will be agreed upon by the committee and the chief executive and will be submitted to the full board for approval 60 days prior to the close of the fiscal year.

Any evaluation factors or standards for performance will be agreed upon in writing at least one year before they are applied in evaluation. The chief executive will meet with the performance evaluation committee and the committee will communicate its findings and feelings while the executive will have opportunity for comments and questions.

If evaluation indicates that the committee feels the executive has not met certain objectives, specific recommendations shall be made for appropriate correction.

Source: Witt Associates Inc.

Consider these questions while you are developing your own policy on CEO evaluation:

— Does the executive know what the board feels about his or her strengths and weaknesses?

— Does the board refrain from criticism in all areas unless it has formally stated its expectations ahead of time?

— Does the board establish a written record of its expectations for both the individual and the organization?

— Does the chief executive have an opportunity to request in writing more direction, support, or resources?

Guidelines for CEO Evaluation

The guidelines for an evaluation always cause a great deal of confusion: Which factors should we use? How shall we weight the factors? Do we need a form? Do we dictate what the factors will be or do we talk with the CEO to establish them? How can we properly evaluate an executive in an industry we know little about? What comparisons with other organizations will give us an adequate barometer of how well our organization and our CEO have done?

Some boards are actually looking for a variation of the Boy Scout oath with its "kind, trustworthy, obedient, brave, clean, and reverent" litany. A board that focuses entirely on those subjective areas may miss the key reason it hired the person in the first place—to get results. The goals or objectives that the board has established must be the central consideration in an evaluation.

Getting Started

As early as 1968 I suggested that factors used will fall into objective and subjective areas. The objective or quantitative areas are easily defined in terms of times, dates, amounts, percentages, ratios, market shares, and so on. The subjective elements are much "softer" and require more discussion. These frequently deal with an individual's style. These changes are much harder to achieve and will take great patience from the board and the CEO.

Two working documents are needed by the performance evaluation committee:

— A current job description for the CEO.
— Written objectives, mutually agreed upon by the board and CEO.

If there is no current job description the committee should direct the CEO to draft one for their discussion and approval. The resulting discussion will be enlightening, and in my opinion it is worth every bit oi the time and effort required. If the committee members agree on the position description, they may present it to the full board for approval.

I've seen boards that took months to get agreement on a definition of the CEO's responsibility. Imagine being the CEO in an organization where everyone on your board has a slightly different view of what you are supposed to be doing! This first step is fundamental and its omission will create a major stumbling block in the evaluation process.

Objectives will take various forms in different businesses.

In some businesses it is simply "to make a profit." Those who have a financial orientation and training may feel that an adequate budget or financial plan is all that's needed in any business. Others may rely on yearly business plans that are made up of both an operating plan and a financial plan.

Committees need to focus on performance as the critical criteria for a CEO appraisal. The board of directors, untrained and uninformed about a highly complex organization such as a hospital when it tries to evaluate the technical competence of a hospital CEO, will have a difficult time. However, if it evaluates whether that individual has accomplished what they agreed upon 12 months ago, the task becomes markedly easier. The board needs to look at broad areas of CEO responsibility to begin its evaluation process.

Results Areas

Not necessarily in rank order, seven broad results areas in which boards may assess the CEO are:

— Consumer needs
— Economic indicators
— Quality
— Productivity
— Personnel development
— Creativity
— Business development

The CEO and board that develop a series of specific objectives in each of these designated results areas will find a great deal to discuss at the annual performance evaluation.

Consumer needs. Too many programs are begun and resources allocated before the board has seen sufficient market research to show what the consumer of health services wants, needs, and is willing to pay for. Health professionals can identify many needs but the question is, what will the public be willing to pay for, at what price, and at what location?

I know hospitals that embarked on ventures in sports medicine, real estate, retirement centers, and wellness. The problem was, the ventures were poorly conceived and not competitively priced, or they were very well received but very unprofitable. Any hospital market area has many needs for services but some of these services are not profitable. Boards need to make sure that all their philanthropic efforts are planned.

Market research is not an extravagant luxury. It is an *investment* in well-planned products and services. It is also a specific way to conserve resources. Unfortunately, many boards pay for the research the hard way, after an unprofitable program is closed.

It would be easy to blame the CEO and the entire management team for these costly errors. But boards that approve programs without sufficient research have to share the responsibility.

Many ventures developed by hospitals in recent years were launched without sufficient hard data. Board members who feel they represent the community ought to make sure they get regular readings from the community. Measuring public needs and wants is essential, and the board that sets goals for management's ability to gather meaningful consumer information in quantifiable form will be well served.

Economic indicators. The most common gauge of success in any business enterprise is the financial statement. Whether the venture is for-profit or non-profit, board members feel comfortable evaluating bottom-line results. But it's not easy to get board agreement on what the financial goals should be. While many cannot agree on whether a bottom-line goal of 3 percent or 15 percent of gross revenue is proper, almost everyone agrees that a deficit is unacceptable.

The vast majority of boards and CEOs have side-stepped a key issue by not targeting the bottom line in their evaluations. The executive with responsibility for a specific percentage increase in revenues or market share will sharpen the focus of his or her management team. The board that succeeds in getting a CEO committed to specific economic results will not wonder how to evaluate him or her at year's end. Market share studies, so common in other industries, will soon add further economic indicators by which to measure the designated results.

Quality. For many years, board members told me the quality of medical care could not be measured. Then, in the 1970s, we watched the development of quality assurance programs and peer review systems, and suddenly we had indicators of quality. Just getting involved in developing standards in these areas was beneficial to the entire industry.

In what other areas can the board direct management to define quality more precisely and then achieve it? The percentage of patients who would recommend your hospital in each category (for example, day-surgery or inpatient) should be 90 percent or above. Survey your physicians annually and determine the degree to which they are satisfied with patient care. If it's not at least 70 percent, I'd say you have work to do. What percentage of clinical departments with quality assurance criteria established are monitoring their effectiveness? What annual reserve for potential claims is funded? What is actually paid out? Have you identified the 5 or 12 or 20 keys to quality service for each department? What objectives does your CEO have to clarify quality issues for the public, employees, medical staff, and management?

Remember that today's market studies constantly show that the general public cannot differentiate between quality or services among hospitals. Any board that hears management and physicians discuss quality knows we need a better definition of terms. Boards that make this a management goal will get not only definition but standards of performance by which to measure quality.

Productivity. This is a designated results area that just cries out for quantification. Even a below-average CEO can produce more with additional people and dollars. What goals does your

CEO set each year to show that productivity relates to organizational effectiveness by departments?

For example, has the CEO established productivity requirements for a large percentage of full-time employees? What percentage of departments have a productivity monitoring system? What percentage of departments have productivity goals that they meet or exceed? What is the departmental full-time equivalent employee cost per hour vs. revenue, and what is the trend?

A wise board will make these measures, ratios, and criteria factors in CEO evaluation. Setting up the criteria is the first goal. After that, progress can be measured in any number of ways. Increased productivity holds valuable potential for any service organization and good CEOs are always willing to have their management teams measured.

Personnel development. Many board members have told me they felt their CEO was surrounded by weak people. How does a board assure itself that managerial ladders are filled with competent, motivated, and growing people? Bench-strength is absolutely essential for the long-term health of the hospital operation. What goals has the CEO established for identifying and training managers?

Someone once wisely stated that only people appreciate in value, while all other assets depreciate. What programs are planned to make your employees more sensitive to the public? To the medical staff? How are you encouraging the most creative and productive individuals to grow within your organization?

A CEO who fosters personnel development can be measured in these ways: Is there a performance appraisal system for all members of management that gives them written objectives as well as annual reports on their results? Is there a program for management development? What are the results? What reward systems have been established for internal personnel development and promotion?

Creativity. During World War II, cash awards were paid for ideas that reduced costs or increased productivity. What is your

CEO doing to see that every person's innovative talents are tapped? Are creativity and new ideas encouraged? How? Are people rewarded? Does the board encourage the CEO to be creative? How do you reward creativity?

The entire health care system has such a rigid pecking order that ideas are frequently buried unless they originate at the top. The CEO who taps the human potential of all the organization's employees can discover amazing resources. What methods are regularly used to give everyone a chance to improve services? What are the rewards? What programs encourage managers to innovate? Is the organization willing to allow some failures to occur?

Every enterprise could be improved if its own people would apply creative thinking to their problems. Boards that stimulate CEOs to use all the possible applied imagination they can will quickly see a ripple effect. Many non-profit atmospheres don't value new ideas, but leadership from the board can have a positive effect in stimulating new thinking.

Business development. This involves the total mission of the institution and its programs. It may entail promotion of specific services or it may result from a base of good will established over generations of service to your community.

What specific programs have been developed to enhance your public image? Your image with the medical staff? Employees? Does the hospital have goals and objectives to make it a responsible corporate citizen? Do you document through public opinion surveys whether your image is better or worse than it was previously?

A Few More Thoughts

The best, most practical way to develop objectives is for the board's executive compensation committee and the CEO to agree on objectives and their priority. The first draft of objectives is prepared by management as a starting point. Weighing the objectives helps both the board and the CEO focus the resources on mutually agreeable areas.

Many variations exist for reporting quarterly progress that show where management responsibility has been delegated and to whom. Some organizations give the levels of achievement for each goal by stating a minimum, optimum, and average result expected. If the projects are complex and require that checkpoints be reached in each quarter, these can be noted.

Look at one successful CEO's management objectives and ask yourself how these goals would satisfy your board. They obviously will change each year according to board directives and organizational needs, but here's a "snapshot" from one organization.

Sample Chief Executive Officer Management Objectives—19XX

The following common management objectives represent desirable future results, expressed in specific terms, to be achieved by the management team during 19XX. They can and will be achieved through the efforts of the chief executive. The board of directors is willing to provide the necessary resources and support. The order of listing is not intended to imply relative importance.

— Achieve an understanding on the part of each member of the management team of the mission statement, the implications of church sponsorship, and the organizational structure of the hospital.

— Begin a formal training program in management.

— Develop a strategic planning process.

— Introduce a corporate hospitality emphasis by training 95 percent of personnel in the importance of courtesy and hospitality, the importance of friendly greetings and the use of names, the importance of personal appearance, and telephone courtesy. Establish an appropriate recognition program to reinforce courteous behavior.

— Establish a physician referral service.

— Achieve understanding by all employed personnel that they must "Dare to Care."

— By responding to the needs of physicians, increase inpatient admissions so that the 19XX total is 3 percent greater than that of the previous year.

— Implement quantitative staffing tools so that hours worked and work-load are closely matched and so that the 19XX operating budget is constructed according to measured staffing needs.

— Improve the decor and appearance of 50 percent of patient and visitor areas where that can be done without extensive remodeling.

— Maintain the implementation schedule for the new information system to the extent possible in the face of uncontrollable software delays, without significant adverse effect on operations.

— Maintain all governmental and regulatory approvals during the year.

— Implement the system of management by objectives at the corporate officer level for 19XX, and establish following year objectives for division directors.

Source: Witt Associates Inc.

If your CEO accomplished every goal on this list, what would be your reaction? What would your response be to the CEO? The challenge for any board is not only to achieve results but to keep the CEO challenged, motivated, and rewarded. The time spent on this process is board work of the most rewarding kind, not some theoretical busy-work project. Try it; you'll like it.

10.

Compensation, Contracts, and Motivation

Boards frequently have problems with executive compensation and benefits. Old stereotypes die hard and people have traditionally felt that non-profit executives are less competent than executives in for-profit enterprises. Board members for years made comparisons with other non-profit or public service executives such as school administrators or elected officials. Hospitals were supposed to be easy to run if you kept the doctors happy and the beds filled in a clean, adequately staffed facility. Those were the days!

In fact, hospitals are among the most complex organizations in any community. Increased competition in the health care marketplace means that organizations must compete for the best talent. Boards soon learn, as one board member stated, "If you pay peanuts, you are liable to get monkeys."

Boards of directors cannot escape the fact that unless executives are fairly compensated, turnover will increase. The cost of replacing a key person is high, and the loss of momentum to the organization and its programs is real. I would estimate that more than three-fourths of new executives are paid more than their predecessors. Therefore, any board should be concerned with attracting, retaining, and motivating key personnel.

Many aspects of this subject are relevant for serious deliberations: What should we pay our executives compared to organizations of similar size and type? How large an area should we include for geographic comparisons? Should compensation issues be handled by the full board or delegated to a committee? Should we establish a formal system or use an ad hoc procedure? What role should incentives play in the overall plan? Should incentives be related to short-term goal achievement or long-term results? What benefits should be provided and why are executives treated any differently? What should be our policy on employment contracts and severance agreements for the CEO and his or her staff? When and if terminations are necessary, what will our policies be for early retirement or temporary relocation assistance? What role will compensation play in the motivation of hospital executives?

What the board does for the CEO will set the tone for what is done for the members of the management team. Executives today understand their worth in the marketplace, and the board must know that what an executive is paid compared to his or her peers affects morale.

Some board members appear to be shocked by the fact that health executives today may earn $250,000 per year or more in salary, plus incentives and benefits. Such persons are running complex institutions with budgets from $150 million to $300 million in annual revenues. In fact, salaries today of $100,000 plus incentives and benefits in organizations with budgets of $30 million to $50 million are classified as routine.

One of the problems most boards face is that only a fraction of most board members earn what the hospital CEO does. For that reason, unless a board is very careful, personal bias rather than objective thought will determine compensation for hospital executives. Lack of objectivity surfaces, particularly when a community or a region has a depressed economy. Board members will rationalize, "We've got to be sensitive to the community," but their first priority had better be to get the best CEO possible. This is where a board's responsibility to corporate mission and purpose requires people who are willing to stand up and be counted.

Philosophy of Compensation

First, boards need to decide at what level they will compensate the CEO and the management team. All sorts of surveys—by size, type, and geographic region—can help a board understand the competitive range for compensation and benefits. The board must decide if it will pay average or above-average salaries. It should be consistent in relating salary level to the performance it expects.

All boards need to review frequently what competing organizations pay. Too often, the accumulation of survey data is left to management, and then the board suspects that the data is biased. To be sure they receive objective information, they must hire compensation consultants who know the health care business and understand the marketplace. Many state association surveys are of little value, in part because they reflect large numbers of people who would not be acceptable as replacements to other boards.

If a board decides to pay its CEO at the 65th percentile, it had better be sure it is getting above-average performance. When the executive performance is disappointing but there are no agreed-upon goals and no understanding of how performance will be measured, it is a real problem. Too often, boards are working with generalizations about performance; the most common measure is last year's performance against the current year's.

Executive Compensation Committees

Boards are best served by appointing a committee to handle all matters related to compensation. This function is more truly board work than most of what boards traditionally do. The executive compensation committee needs people who have had experience with executive compensation and benefits, if at all possible. People who understand compensation and benefits will treat the matter professionally. Usually, three members are sufficient.

A word of caution: Some board members who lack perspective may zero in on executive pay as an issue the whole board must discuss. I have actually seen boards with a $40 million budget spend hours discussing whether a 10 percent raise in base salary is too generous for the CEO. Compensation issues are not the whole board's business; let a committee handle it.

Once again, the best foundation for any committee is a written statement of purpose: The general function of the executive compensation committee is to ensure that the executive compensation practices of the organization are competitive with the national marketplace, allowing the organization to attract, retain, motivate, and reward the most competent executive and managerial talent available.

Some board members may want comparative data only from local competitive institutions. That is not realistic. When replacing executives, organizations do not limit their search to the local market. No committee should ever apologize for paying top dollar to get the best talent available. Quite the contrary—I have never seen the public or the press congratulate a board for *thriftiness* in hiring average or below-average people for key positions. If the board wants to launch a cost-control effort, the CEO's salary is a poor place to start.

After the executive compensation committee understands its basic function, the members might have specific duties such as the following:

— Establish the institution's executive compensation and benefits philosophy.
— Conduct the performance appraisal of the CEO.
— Keep informed on current national health care executive compensation trends.

— Establish the executive salaries budget and adjustments annually.

— Approve all executive compensation policies.

— Establish fringe benefits and perquisites that maximize benefit dollars for the institution and the individual receiving them.

— Negotiate any employment contract or severance agreements with key executives.

— Administer any executive incentive programs.

— Retain outside counsel as necessary to assist in development of the executive compensation programs.

— Define an annual meeting schedule and agenda topics.

The specific duties will vary from one organization to another, but appraisal of the CEO's performance should be a vital concern for this committee. I have found after years of recommending the committee concept that initially, few organizations disagree; but a year later, few had met or knew how to begin. Some wonder if there is enough work for a committee. I suggest an annual agenda for an executive compensation committee. The following sample assumes that committee activities from year to year follow the institution's fiscal year, which is identical to the calendar year.

Sample Agendas for Executive Compensation Committee

Meeting 1:   January

1. Appraise the CEO's performance, objectives, and achievements.
2. Review and adjust compensation ranges or benefits as necessary.
3. Establish objectives for the year.
4. Any other committee business.

Meeting 2:   April

1. Review the CEO's report on the executive performance of his or her immediate subordinates.
2. Discuss incentive compensation and review at least three comparably sized organizations' plans.
3. Detail any requests for further information needs of the committee.
4. Review first quarter's progress on objectives.

Meeting 3:   September

1. Review consultant's compensation survey and decide on any changes necessary.
2. Review second quarter's progress on objectives for the year.
3. Any other committee business.

Meeting 4:   November

1. Review third-quarter progress on objectives.
2. Review first draft of objectives for the coming year.
3. Approve and forward confidential executive salary and benefits amounts for the next annual budget.
4. Any other committee business.

Starting this process is the hardest part. Once the process is under way, it will change and improve to provide the necessary give-and-take for meaningful communication. As the process becomes familiar, it will help everyone concerned. Done well, it will require time, effort, and deliberation, but there should be fewer surprises for both parties at year's end.

Establishing Objectives

Compensation always relates to performance. When targets are hit, goals are reached and exceeded, any executive will expect more than a cost-of-living adjustment. If goals are not achieved, targets missed, and results less than satisfactory, the committee will have to decide about minimum adjustments, no adjustments, or even termination. However, some failures in organizational efforts will not be due to lack of effort but to forces outside the control of management.

The board must sign off on management's goals and objectives for the coming year or determine its own priorities for management. In some hospitals, the CEO prepares a summary of all the goals and objectives in a single three- or four-page report for the committee. Committee members may offer suggestions and changes, but once they have adopted the report, it becomes the action plan for the year. One year later the committee reviews performance on the goals and objectives previously agreed upon.

In other organizations, the board prepares a broad "wishlist" of achievements for the organization, in keeping with its mission statement. The CEO and management team prepare their list. After discussion, the two lists are melded together to become the business plan for the year. Some boards heavily weight their lists with a specific bottom-line figure, a control-of-expenses factor, a business-increase factor, a market research goal, a physician-mix plan, and an admitting-improvement factor for each staff member. The direction and nature of the list give management a picture of what the board expects. Do they always hit all the targets? No, but the process works well.

Base Salaries

What is a fair base salary? When does a board pay more than average? Is it ever possible to pay less than average? What is a fair adjustment or an annual raise for a CEO or key management executive? Are base salaries related to incentives or bonuses? Do you need a formal salary structure? These are some of the questions board members ask when considering this subject. Pat answers are not possible, but let's explore the broad issue.

Most boards want to be fair as well as competitive. Failure to be competitive means that a board accepts its role as a stepping stone for people who will leave for better-paying positions. The board must approve a reasonable salary structure for the CEO and his or her immediate subordinates. This means that each position should have a salary range with minimums and maximums to help a board objectively review where the organization is vis-à-vis comparable institutions. Internal equity is another benefit.

If a board is promoting internally, it may be able to pay a below-average rate as someone learns the ropes and proves that he or she can handle the additional responsibility. When a person who is untested as a CEO moves in from outside the organization, the pay may be average or above. When the board seeks to attract an experienced CEO, the hospital's current salary range will not be as significant a factor as the desired candidate's current base salary.

For example, an executive in a $40 million organization with seven years of experience as a successful CEO is currently making $100,000 in base salary. For that individual to give up the known position he has for the unknown may require a 25 or 30 percent improvement factor, assuming that living costs and other factors are fairly equal. Thus, $130,000 would be a fair offer. A board should never let $5,000 or $10,000 deny them their choice of a new CEO.

Annual adjustments are another matter. Usually, these are keyed to the adjustment given to the total work force, or to the cost of living. When a CEO achieves goals established by their board, 5 to 7 percent in addition to the cost of living is not an unreasonable annual adjustment. In some places, the same percentage added to what the total work force receives would be considered fair. This assumes the CEO is in a competitive salary range. What if the CEO is at the maximum? Then annual adjustments would match general adjustments. If the CEO is still young and mobile and has had two or three years of little or no adjustment, the board may need to look at incentives if they want to keep the CEO motivated.

Because of the political nature of most hospitals, few CEOs will work 30 years at one institution. As institutions merge, consolidate, and sell out, loyalty becomes hard for a board to reward. Nevertheless, as a board seeks to make its organization grow, prosper, or survive, it will want to keep competent executives as long as it can.

Incentives

In for-profit organizations, various methods are used to keep executives motivated. Many of these link pay to performance. Common examples of these are bonuses, deferred bonus plans, stock options, incentive stock options, stock appreciation rights, phantom stock, and a host of variations on these themes.

These methods can be divided into two broad categories: short-term incentives and long-term incentives. Most hospital board members will ask what that has to do with hospitals, and the answer increasingly is—plenty. As hospital executives are pushed to win the competitive wars for dollars with their economic peers, the winners want more than generous merit increases.

Meanwhile, in the last few years board members have increasingly looked to incentives as partial alternatives to compensation adjustments. They feel (somewhat inappropriately, in my opinion) that an incentive system will make adjustments easier. This is only partially true, as the judgment factors are seldom removed from any incentive plan.

Short-term plans are usually designed to provide bonuses for a single year's efforts. They are paid within a few months after the conclusion of the year. Usually, they are stated as a percentage of base salary, generally 15 to 30 percent of base for the executive group.

For this discussion, *executive group* is approximately equal to 0.5 percent of the total employee group. Therefore, in a small hospital with 300 or fewer employees, we are only speaking of one or two people, while the 1,000-employee institution will have five to eight key executives.

Long-term incentives, which are preferred by for-profit boards, are rewards for performance accomplishments over a period of several years. Because shareholders and investors want their dollars to grow, long-term executive incentives are tied to increases in shareholder dollars. Thus, an executive who is hired as CEO or marketing vice-president when the company's stock sells for $20 per share may be given options for 1,000 shares of that stock, payable after three or five years. If, three years later, the stock is selling for $40 per share, the executive who helped investors double the value of their investment gets a chance to share the wealth.

As hospitals have recently experimented with incentives, the majority are using short-term incentives to pay bonuses. The longer those plans are in effect, the more boards will tie performance to long-term incentives. However imperfect the systems are, I estimate that 40 to 50 percent of all hospital executives will be covered by various forms of short-term and long-term incentives by the early 1990s.

Executive Benefits

This is an interesting area affected by three variables: general benefits for all employees, competitive benefits provided for comparable executives in similar-size organizations, and status symbols.

A long time ago, every hospital employee got the same benefits, including health insurance, pension, vacation, and holidays, until it became apparent that this all-employees-are-equal idea was nonsense. Everyone knows that for-profit and non-profit executives are treated exactly like professional baseball managers. When the team wins, "Hurray for our genius manager, that crafty fox!" When the team loses, we seldom trade the players or remove the bat boy, we replace the manager.

All employees are not equal. We pay some more than others. Executives regularly arrive early and work late. Weekend duty is commonplace. And when they recommend a course of action to the board and it proves to be wrong, they find it very hard to hide. Improved benefits partially compensate for the extra pressures, responsibilities, and burdens.

Some benefits protect executive income. A supplemental retirement policy for a given executive may cost $10,000. If that executive is in a 50 percent tax bracket and paid for the policy with his or her own funds, he or she would need to receive $20,000 as compensation; but if the organization paid, it would be half that expense.

This same idea applies to the development of deferred compensation plans, disability income, and supplemental life insurance. The latest changes in tax laws mean there will be a new bundle of executive benefits conceived by consultants, accountants, and attorneys. It is part of the worldwide recognition that rank will have its privileges.

It is easy to justify many benefits and perquisites. These were the benefits listed for CEOs in a recent Witt Associates survey. Not all are received by everyone, but the list offers some food for thought.

Benefits Received by CEO
Car
Gas credit card
Repairs and maintenance
Country club membership
Luncheon/town club dues
Entertainment credit card
Spouse travel
First-class travel
Health club dues
Annual physical
Financial planning

Legal counsel
Professional dues
Low-interest loans
Pharmacy discount
Tuition discount
Educational assistance

Source: *The Witt Report*, Volume II, April 1986

It is easy to understand the provision of a car to an executive traveling to and from meetings. If you provide the car, then funds to keep it running are only proper maintenance of the original investment. Membership in country clubs and luncheon clubs always sounds lavish, but in fact they can be useful if you want the key hospital executives to socialize amidst the local power structure. Many meetings for board, medical staff, and management are also held in such facilities. As you look at the list, it is easy to see how these benefits can be included in the total compensation package of most executives. These benefits are viewed initially as a prize, and later as a right.

Contracts

This phenomenon has clearly developed the last few years because of all the changes, pressures, and uncertainties in health care. Most new CEOs today ask for and receive a contract. This trend will spread to other key positions as well. In 1984, Witt Associates published a booklet of sample contracts entitled *Contracts For Health Care Executives*. Boards need to be aware that contracts that protect a CEO may also protect the board.

The three common types of agreements mentioned in that book were the employment contract, the protective covenant, and the senior consultant contract.

Employment contract. This is prepared at the time the executive is hired. It usually states the salary, goals to be achieved, and when and how performance toward those goals will be reviewed. It also usually guarantees employment for a specified period of time, barring major disasters, and provides a severance agreement guaranteeing that the terminated executive will receive salary and benefits for a designated period of time, except in extreme cases.

Protective covenant. A protective covenant is given to the current CEO who is asked to take significant new risks, such as terminating an impaired physician, or merging one hospital with another.

In these risky situations, it is possible that board members would bend (and some have done so) to the pressures of the media, community, or medical staff, with the result that another CEO loses his position. In fairness to all parties, a protective covenant offers the gentleman's way out. It assures that the CEO will not become a "sacrificial lamb" and it protects the institution from taking action casually.

Senior consultant contract. Finally, the senior consultant contract is useful in the final five or so years prior to retirement. It is designed to provide good-faith rewards to the practicing, older CEO while protecting the institution on a long-range basis. It spells out the salary and benefits for the retiring CEO while defining the transition of the successor CEO. Thus, transition can become a planned, scheduled event rather than an interim crisis. The institution, the current CEO, and the successor all benefit from the agreement, as the obligations and responsibilities of each are clearly stated.

Terminations

This process is unpleasant, but it can be helpful to all parties if it is done fairly and honestly. Granted, some executives are shown the door and asked to leave for good reasons. However, the majority depart with real accomplishments and the potential to help another organization.

It used to be a strong negative to have been fired, but the

whole process needs rethinking today. Lee Iacocca is the best example I know of. Henry Ford's effort to penalize Iacocca became the lifeboat Chrysler needed for its very survival. An interesting book by Richard Gould, *Why Good People Get Fired,* points out that under-performance is *not* the biggest reason people get terminated. Most terminations occur for hospital CEOs because of a change in board philosophy. The board that hires a CEO is seldom the one that fires him. Often, a new board with a different chairperson and philosophy finds it difficult to work with the CEO.

In other cases, boards that realized in the first year that they made a mistake in hiring or promoting the CEO may have left the termination to a succeeding group of board members.

An integrative process for termination would include an economic settlement and the offer to the executive of outplacement services. This is simply a humanitarian approach to an otherwise messy situation. Outplacement and a settlement will allow executives the time to reevaluate their circumstances and to make logical plans to rebuild their careers.

Many board members ask how much severance is reasonable. Just for discussion purposes, I've related tenure to the suggested amount of severance in the chart on the facing page.

Motivation

Hospital boards seldom see their role as motivators of the CEO. They may feel the CEO should fire *them* up for *their* job. However, the board's role is clearly to direct and motivate the executive in terms of what they expect, and then assure themselves that the CEO is moving decisively to accomplish the agreed-upon goals. If an executive is constantly wondering how he or she is doing, whether the board is pleased, or what faction of the medical staff opposes him or her, the effect is draining.

Any board wants a confident executive leading the hospital's employees, pioneering new programs, and causing growth and long-term benefits to the future health of the organization.

Years of Salary Severance
Related to Tenure

Tenure	5	10	15	20	30
Age					
	2	2	3	4	5
60					
	1	2	3	4	4
55					
	1	2	3	3	4
50					
	1	2	2	3	3
45					
	1	1	2	2	3
40					

Find your CEO's age and cross with his or her years of tenure. For example, the 60-year-old CEO with 14 years of tenure should receive at least three years of salary as severance.

When a board treats its CEO as an equal or better, provides economic rewards related to performance, and has a no-fault economically secure conclusion to the relationship (should that become necessary), the CEO will have no excuse for not producing.

A board may be conservative in many areas, but in trying to ensure that its executive team is charged up, it will be wise to be generous while expecting above-average results. Such a board will never be at fault if the organization fails. And it can claim a major share of credit when it succeeds.

11.

Working with the Medical Staff

The preceding chapters have all dealt with the internal, board-centered issues that every board of directors has to confront and process successfully. This chapter acknowledges that there is a world outside the boardroom, and specifically a world inhabited by those strange and fabulous creatures called the medical staff. In no other board situation would you be called upon to deal with such an unusual group—neither employee nor freelance consultant, but nonetheless an integral part of the hospital mechanism.

Fasten your seatbelts—it's going to be a bit bumpy here.

The most sensitive relationship in a hospital organization is that between the board of directors and the medical staff. The attitude of the board, and its understanding of the medical staff organization (MSO) and individual physicians, are critical factors in this relationship.

Boards view physicians as employees, technicians, entrepreneurs, or business people, and a few board members hold physicians with the reverence normally reserved for major deities. But physicians are *not* employees; they are agents of the organization. These physician-agents act in cooperation with the hospital as independent contractors.

Many new hospital board members mistakenly assume that the hospital can direct and control all physicians as it would any employee. When physicians see patients in their offices, they are truly independent professionals. When they are granted privileges on a hospital medical staff and bring their patients to the hospital, they are theoretically loosely controlled and directed by the self-governing process of the medical staff organization. That process is very much misunderstood by board members today.

The board of directors is responsible for quality patient services in the institution. Legally and morally, the board is responsible for inviting only competent physicians to practice at the hospital. The medical staff's responsibility is to assure the board of their professionalism. Boards must depend on these physicians to act as their advisors in areas where they lack technical knowledge and skill.

When the physicians as independent contractors form an organized body with bylaws it is because they are affiliated with the hospital and responsible to its board. A medical staff does not organizationally exist if it is not affiliated with and subordinate to a hospital board. Board members quickly learn that only rarely does the collective medical staff have a unified opinion on *anything*. Many individual physicians may speak long and loud on a cause dear to their own hearts and say, "This is how the *whole* staff feels," but experience has shown that is very unlikely.

Ordering physicians around as if they were employees will not work and board members soon learn this fact. Power plays usually result in standoffs between boards and medical staffs that slow the hospital's accomplishment of its corporate purpose.

The quality of the hospital is inextricably tied to the composition of the medical staff and the quality of the physicians who are admitted to practice there. Board members must recognize their own roles in medical staff appointments, quality assurance, staff recruitment, staff discipline, and replacement. Building a constructive relationship between a board and a medical staff is a fundamental goal for all excellent hospitals. A board that allows its medical stafi to do as it pleases will reap the same rewards as the parents of a spoiled child. A board that fights its medical staff or is politically maneuvered by them is headed straight for mediocrity, or worse.

A Historical Perspective on Physicians

To understand physicians today, one needs to appreciate the past. Until the 1920s, physicians were not held in the highest esteem. Hard to believe, but true. "Quack" and "sawbones" were not affectionate terms; they expressed how people sometimes felt about physicians in an earlier day. Rural Americans and immigrants in cities could not afford routine medical treatment. People did not seek out hospitals or physicians except in critical situations. Physician quality varied widely, depending on where the physician had been trained.

However, U.S. medical education took a quantum leap forward with the publication in 1910 of the Flexner report. Abraham Flexner, an educator, was appointed by the Carnegie Foundation to evaluate public, private, and proprietary medical schools. At that time, the country had an oversupply of poorly trained physicians. The public's distrust of physicians was justified, based on the lack of uniformity in their training. Standards to separate the good from the bad were lacking. Self-policing by groups such as the American Medical Association was politically impossible. The basic effect of the Flexner report was to limit the number of medical schools and their graduates. Once standards for laboratories, libraries, and faculties were established, weak organizations were forced to spend the time and money to comply, or close their doors. The pendulum swung toward uniform accreditation for quality medical education, and the overall quality of medicine in the U.S. was raised.

As more standardized medical education and training became the norm, hospitals became an integral part of the whole scheme. Hospital internships created strong ties between physicians and hospitals. Hospitals near medical schools quickly aligned with those schools to provide themselves credibility. Hospital boards quickly attempted to provide facilities for training physicians.

Eventually, private practicing physicians and those in academic medicine became two separate camps, not always friendly or compatible. The difference in motivation is apparent to those who work with one or the other type of physician. Both groups are interested in power. Faculty members get power from appointments and the status of university positions. During the last 30 years, those in private practice have established their power and position by their ability to earn high incomes, independent of corporate control.

Legally, only physicians can admit patients to hospitals. This means doctors' admitting patterns can greatly affect an institution's financial position. Such economic clout is clearly used in confrontations between a board and its medical staff. While physicians may not be unified often, any perceived threat to their economic well-being can generate great consensus.

After World War II, the real split between those two camps of physicians grew quickly, furthered by the emergence of medical specialties. The technology developed for field hospitals and facilities for specialists created a sad fallout—a competitive game among hospitals to see who could attract the most specialists. Gadgetry on a grand scale attracted young physicians who were eager to let new technologies establish their credibility. Hospital after hospital upgraded its facilities, and medical staffs pressured their hospital boards to provide funds for the latest facilities and equipment. The Hill-Burton legislation of the 1950s offered all communities the funds to build or upgrade hospitals. The race was on, and every board had a building committee.

The growing post-war population, the expanding suburbs, and the shortage of hospital beds caused physicians to seek staff privileges at more than one hospital. It was not uncommon for specialists to have privileges at three or four hospitals and to use two of those hospitals regularly. Very quickly, doctors learned to put pressure on several boards at once to provide facilities. The silent threat to all boards was, "Unless you provide the beds and technology here, we will take our patients to the neighboring hospital." Hospitals concerned about physician shortages made sure they had all the latest diagnostic gizmos.

Most hospital boards acknowledged these economic statements: "To fill our beds, we need physicians. To have a high occupancy rate, we have to keep the doctors happy." That simplistic equation led boards to base all their organizational philosophies for dealing with individual physicians and the medical staff organization on keeping doctors happy. Although boards of directors have always had a legal and moral responsibility for quality care and for eliminating excessive hospital stays, it wasn't until the government mandated regulations that the board began to do its job.

Understanding Physicians

Until about 1960, the dominant work model for physicians was private practice. They left medical school, hung out their shingle, and began to see patients. Post-World War II physicians were accepted as miracle workers with independence and professional esteem. They provided the cure and patients covered by insurance and prepayment did not have to be concerned about the cost. Doctors didn't always enjoy enough financial success, but building a practice was thought to be a career-long proposition.

Physicians were taught to act and think in terms of the patient. No part of the medical school curriculum included learning how to work in organizations, how organizations functioned, or why cost control and management skills were necessary. These issues are still not formally addressed in most medical schools. Despite the fact that the majority of physicians leaving medical school today do not want solo practice, most medical education still prepares people for the independence of their own shingle. Today, the majority of young physicians prefer the security of salaries and group affiliations, but their training hasn't caught up with the real world.

Specialization had a profound effect on physicians and how the public perceived them. If the family physician needed a population base of 1,000 to 3,000 to support his or her practice, that practice could be established in a small town or in a neighborhood in a large city. Such a doctor felt that knowledge about patients' family histories was a necessary ingredient to establishing a practice. Specialists, on the other hand, needed a much larger population base. The pediatric neurologist might require a base of 100,000 to 300,000, for example, to support a practice. This meant that people traveled long distances to see specialists who did not know the family history, who in fact had limited opportunity to learn what they believed to be extraneous information. The extended training required of the specialists delayed their opportunity to earn an income. Once out in practice, however, their higher fees seemed justified to their peers as well as to their patients.

All physicians endured their years of training because they valued having financial independence and freedom from organizational constraints. It is no accident that suburbs of major cities never experienced physician shortages. Physicians located their offices where people had the ability to pay for their services, and avoided places where the general population lacked the ability to pay. Attorneys and accountants make similar choices for similar reasons.

While it's important to understand where we came from, it is now necessary to update our current perceptions in terms of today's world. Board members need to understand the changing patterns not only of hospital but also of medical practices.

Boards need to see clearly that physician's incomes and professional competence depend on the hospitals they practice in. Just as attorneys need courts to earn their incomes if they practice law, physicians need hospitals. The mutuality of interests of both doctors and hospitals is therefore well established in our society. Today, boards must understand their obligation to oversee physicians, being neither too strict nor too lax. Leaning too far forward or backward can disturb the balance that is essential to control, and can lead to polarization between a board and medical staff.

Some boards are overwhelmed by the idea of overseeing professionals when they have little or no understanding of medical science. But think—in a democratic society, we allow some very average people to be elected to offices that oversee complex bureaucracies. We also allow trained professionals in our military to report to civilian appointees. The fact is, boards need to see this responsibility as a part of the job. Objectivity and common sense are more necessary for this function than is a knowledge of medicine.

Medical Staff Organization

The medical staff organization is an anomaly in a logical, businesslike organization. Theoretically, at least, the MSO exists to provide an internal government system for a group of professional peers. In fact, it is almost a "shadow" organization that must be acknowledged for its power and influence.

Most organizations will fit within the geometric shape of a triangle.

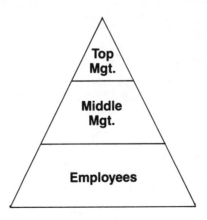

Hospital organizations can be simplified to fit in that same shape. However, there is a parallel organizational structure that overlaps—the medical staff organization.

This side-by-side organization could be illustrated as follows:

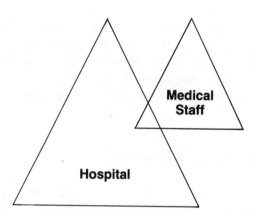

Both of these structures in turn might be overlaid by a larger triangle whose apex would be the governing body that oversees both the management and medical staff organizational structures, if that is actually the case. This is shown in the illustration on the facing page.

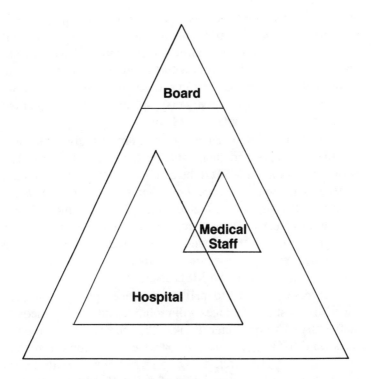

Most boards will need to better understand the purpose of the medical staff organization. How does the MSO support the hospital and its corporate purpose? What responsibilities does the MSO have? How often are those responsibilities evaluated? If responsibilities are not being met, what procedure is followed to correct that condition? What if the staff officers' responsibilities are not clearly supportive of the institution's mission and goals? What if the medical staff's responsibilities are not defined?

Medical practitioners are all members of the MSO. They elect officers from among their peers. In large MSOs, there will be breakdowns by medical specialties with elected department chairpersons. Effectiveness in the MSO is directly related to those officers and their capabilities. A real problem occurs in many MSOs because there are few, if any, specifications for staff leadership. Some voluntary elected department heads or staff leaders are qualified, interested, and dedicated to coordinating the staff efforts with the hospital's own strategic plans. Other people in the same hospital organization, however, may not want to serve, may not be interested, or may avoid decisions and create problems.

Few boards set management or administrative standards for MSO officers and then evaluate their effectiveness. The board may want the MSO to be acting in unison when, in fact, its leaders are consensus-seekers rather than leaders. MSOs are seldom cohesive, well-directed units. They are more like a federation of causes than a corporation. Individual members take great pride in their independence. Rare is the MSO that disciplines one of its members for disloyalty to the hospital, hospital personnel, or the MSO itself.

Perceived threats to private practice, physicians' prerogatives, or staff privileges will mobilize and solidify medical staff unity. The physician thinks, "If they can limit another physician's privileges, income, or style today, tomorrow they can limit me." This circle-the-wagons mentality usually forces a lockstep vote by the majority of the staff. Many a hospital CEO has been terminated by a vocal 20 percent of the medical staff while 80 percent said nothing.

Other issues will polarize the medical staff along economic and social lines. If, for example, the family practitioners are debating an issue with hospital management, the board should not be surprised that surgeons will take the family practice side. Understanding the issues is not as important as understanding where surgeons get their referrals. The same will be true for other economic or professional alliances that exist without benefit of organization charts. Be respectful of the economic alliances first, then the social bonds, and finally, the issues themselves. The same phenomenon can be observed in a staff with many foreign medical school graduates. Watch how they band together on issues as a block.

One suggestion is for boards to strengthen themselves by preparing a written director job description, establishing board standards of performance, developing a job description for the chairperson, and developing a performance appraisal mechanism for the CEO. Accomplishing those basic elements would earn the respect of the MSO. When a board does not have its own act together, it usually must accept whatever performance is offered. Most MSOs could profit from studying and developing some of the same guidelines that apply to boards.

Any board member who hopes to work with an MSO must understand its tradition as well as its strengths and weaknesses. When the board seeks to make an MSO effective instead of merely ceremonial, it can unlock unlimited potential for improvement.

Corporate Practice and Private Practice

Most board members retain a stereotype of the rugged individualist physician. However, young physicians today look for opportunities to practice in groups, clinics, and other corporate structures. Rarely do individuals in today's economic condition decide to go into solo practice.

Some hospital boards wanted to open satellite hospitals and clinics 15 years ago, but their medical staff opposed what might have been good corporate strategy for the hospital. The opposition was seldom based on the economic issues; rather, physicians opposed competition on the grounds that it was corporate practice of medicine. Many boards today still seek to compete with and please their physicians at the same time. Boards are asking their CEOs to find alternate income due to their declining inpatient census. The push is on to get a larger share of the public's health care dollar. At the same time, physicians are also trying to replace their shrinking incomes. Thus, every move made by a hospital manager to take dollars from physicians is a real threat. Boards have to remember their obligation is to the hospital organization and its long-term mission of growth and survival.

Consider the emergency room (ER). Until about 1970, responsible community hospitals required all active members of the MSO to take a turn on call for ER duty. It was understood that this volunteer service was to offset the privilege of using the community hospital for their patients. But people used their insurance and prepayment systems in the hospital emergency rooms when they could not find an open doctor's office on weekends or nights and overloaded the system. The voluntary staffing of large urban ERs collapsed under this increased use of the hospital service.

That collapse led to the emergence of full-time ER groups (again, private practices not physician employees) who served the hospital's emergency room 24 hours a day, seven days a week. Now, we have a subspecialty of physicians who set up corporations and are given a monopoly to cover the ERs of one or more hospitals. What once was voluntary has become a paid position.

Physicians in private practice have to survive and prosper. That is how they pay their rent, pay office personnel salaries, and make their own livings. Hospital boards need to understand, therefore, that physicians have a business motivation, as well as any possible altruistic motives. Strategic plans of the hospital that require physician involvement should ensure that physicians and the hospital both get their economic motives on the table very early. Hospital strategies in competitive areas that presuppose physician involvement would probably serve all parties best if they were contractual.

The board must never forget that its obligation is to the well-being of the hospital corporation. Keeping it economically sound and strategically positioned is vital to its continued existence. While every effort should be made to cooperate with loyal physicians, boards need to realize that some necessary decisions will not be popular with physicians.

Hospital-Based Physicians

These are the specialists who generally earn the majority of their income from a practice based in the hospital. They are granted a monopoly to provide services, such as radiology, pathology, anesthesia, or emergency medical care. For years, many radiologists and pathologists contracted with hospitals to be paid a percentage of gross departmental revenue. Some of these same groups then opened private labs across the street, *in direct competition* with the hospital. All in the spirit of free enterprise, of course.

In the last ten years, many hospital-based physician groups have moved to separate billing arrangements. Board members should know, therefore, that there are *two* businesses providing services and billing to the same patient. Any board that grants a monopoly to the hospital-based physicians should always understand how much competition it has allowed to develop and then frequently assess its own competitive role.

As recently as 1984, a board member in a large Eastern hospital told me he saw no problem with the hospital's pathologists operating a private lab in the hospital's own physician office building across the street! When it was pointed out that the hospital pathology department's revenue was down 15 percent and that five pathology employees had left in one year to join the private lab, that board member still didn't see the problem. When asked if he would see any problem if his company's sales manager worked nights and weekends as an independent sales representative for a competitor, he said he thought that would definitely not be right. Amazing, but true!

Stereotypes die hard. Many board members feel that physicians are their allies because they share patients and sell them services. In some instances they may be, but members of a hospital's medical staff also are competing for patients' dollars. In the last few years, much has been said about cooperation between hospitals and their medical staffs. Boards need to remember that there is a fine line between cooperation and appeasement. If the hospital's economic well-being is sacrificed for political calm, its future could be in jeopardy.

Future Physician Roles

The game is changing, however, and three factors will influence the future of physicians and hospitals: the increasing supply of physicians in all specialties; the continued pressure from health maintenance organizations (HMOs), government, insurance companies, and employers, to cap or control fees; and a tendency for physicians to seek salaries and economic security rather than independent practice with all its pressures. These interrelated developments will create new problems for physicians and the hospitals where they work.

As greater numbers of physicians become available, hospital boards will need to review all the policies and strategies that were deeply rooted in fears of a perpetual shortage. Like the poor widow with five children who wins the big lottery, some changes in strategy are now necessary.

More hospitals will seek to hire physicians as full-time employees to staff new and existing programs. Younger physicians will opt for economic security rather than the independence that was valued by their predecessors. Those hospitals that structure their compensation plans to reward physicians correctly will provide total health care with a full-time staff of professionals under one corporate organization. Physicians have historically looked to private practice to allow them the freedom to work as hard as they wanted and earn as much as they desired. Protection of private practice is not included in any institutional mission statement I've ever seen, however.

Competition in any team sport requires that all players submit to the direction and strategy of the coach. The hospital that can provide all the opportunities for financial and professional growth under its corporate umbrella will win most consistently. Those organizations that assume we can preserve the same voluntary cooperation that existed in the non-competitive era of the 1950s and 1960s may be whistling in the dark. Competition is the tool that the government, the public, and large purchasers of health care have decided to use to control health care costs.

When a large clinic or group practice controls one institution, it has the same effect because the control that is necessary for a "team effort" is present. Many examples exist in the last few years of a hospital MSO fighting the hospital's formation of an HMO, only to have a sizable percentage of that same MSO later join one that is controlled by an organization *com-*

peting with the hospital. Board members need to keep their minds open to the new world, which may include new organizational structures.

12.

The Rewards of Service

To close this book without discussing the rewards
of board service would be an injustice to the more than 50,000
people who serve on hospital boards. The job is difficult and
growing more complex all the time, yet these men and women
accept the responsibility. Why?

As I see it, the tradition of service on these voluntary
boards goes back to town meetings in colonial America. Volunteers have always been a driving force in our country's history. Our governmental system was conceived with public
service as an integral part of the democratic process. Our
churches and fraternal orders founded many organizations with
the primary mission of social service.

Why People Serve on Boards

At the turn of the century President Theodore Roosevelt
said something like, "The mark of an educated person is his or

her willingness to give something back to society." Almost a century before, President John Adams stated it another way: "Public service is the mark of an enlightened electorate."

That question—why people serve on boards—was asked routinely in a questionnaire that I have used for many years in board seminars throughout the country. The aggregate responses provide a meaningful list of the real rewards of board service as seen by board members themselves.

Satisfaction. Many people accept the responsibility because board service does offer many satisfactions. When the organization they oversee pioneers new programs, for example, it vicariously gives board members an experience similar to that of Jonas Salk, when he developed the vaccine for polio. Helping others can give you a big kick, no doubt about it.

Involvement. Some people say they prefer not to sit on the sidelines as a spectator; they want to be involved with the strategies and policies that create and sustain life-saving programs. Those people who have multiple board experiences often characterize this feeling of being involved as a real emotional lift.

Getting to know your community. Because hospitals are concerned with so many aspects of life, their board members must constantly be learning about community needs, resources, problems, and solutions. Board members who have served for long periods of time find that this is especially rewarding.

Making a contribution. Contributing time, effort, support, or expertise is a real reward. Many people derive great satisfaction from merely being present at every meeting to observe and listen. Other people who have special expertise are most rewarded when they are called on to use those special talents in specific task forces and committees. The contribution can be large or small, but making it is valued by board members.

Learning. This is listed as a reason for serving most often by new board members, who feel that learning how a governing body is organized and how it functions is a reward in itself. Board members with the inclination to learn about social issues, political affairs, or new medical technologies can often satisfy their curiosity through their service.

Leadership skills development. A certain number of people presume that if the board is "running the organization," then the board must be a group of leaders. The assumption may be incorrect, but it is a fact that the best known board members in industry often agree to serve on a board just to see another CEO's style of leadership. If board members feel that an opportunity to develop their leadership skills is available, the reward is very real.

Gaining respect. Women whose husbands are busy and successful in their own worlds may feel a real need to establish their own identity. Board service can do that. Another group that has frequently listed this point consists of people whose occupation does not gain them much respect, although it may have gained them financial independence. For example, a plumbing contractor on one board recalled that, because of his sometimes messy appearance, he felt inferior in social situations. Such persons can and do contribute greatly, and their special reward is the respect they get as successful business people.

Prestige or status. Most people will admit that being on the board has more psychological reward than doing a door-to-door canvass for an organization or other grunt-work tasks. It is also one of the reasons why hospital letterheads for years contained all the board members' names. When people are asked to serve on two boards they will usually opt for the one they feel has the most status. The financial scope of most hospitals alone offers board members more opportunity for status than any other not-for-profit activity in their communities.

Recognition. Without question this is a powerful incentive for people to serve on a hospital board. People feel they have "arrived" if they are asked to serve on a board. The social structure of most communities is a very real arena, and being asked to serve on the board indicates a genuine acceptance at the highest levels.

Direct financial rewards. Some boards pay their directors fees for their service. I'm not talking about a clandestine, pocket-lining scheme, but about those institutions that have an appropriately established policy for director compensation. However, most directors who meet all the qualifications have sufficient means so that financial rewards are not the primary reason anyone accepts director responsibilities.

Indirect financial rewards. These are the equivalent of executive "perks" for board members. Some board members attend every convention of their state and national hospital association, no matter where they are held. They view the paid travel and expenses as a reward for their board efforts. Rank does have its privileges. Other hospital board members enjoy hospital discounts for services received and value this benefit highly. The indirect rewards are varied, but very real.

Association with community-minded people. This factor is particularly strong in medium-sized cities where I've personally seen some of the best boards in operation. The hospital board in one such city had only nine members, but they were the presidents of the nine largest employers in that community. It was truly an elite group and the hospital was the only place they all worked together. If powerful people sit on your board, it may be very gratifying for other members.

Fiduciary responsibility. This may either be the personal interest of a financial executive, or simply one interest of the corporate executive who is on the hospital board because his superior wants him there, to watch health care costs. One labor leader in a governmentally owned but privately leased facility stated, "I'm here to guard the henhouse."

Learning about a new business. Health care is like no other business in town. Some board members are intellectually challenged by that fact, so much so that they switch fields and move full-time into the business because of the exposure they've had as board members. I know personally of more than 20 board members who have developed health care consulting practices, lucrative full-time positions, or thriving part-time businesses because of their board experience and contacts.

Interest in health care. Some people who early in life thought of nursing or medicine, but who never took that fork in the road, are attracted to service for this reason. In later life they may feel the strong pull of the compassion exemplified in health care. Others have been deeply touched by what a hospital's health care team did for a parent or family member and now they want to do their part to be of service. Some of the most devoted, loyal board members I've met have strong emotional stories to tell about what keeps them on a hospital board.

Civic or religious duty. Someone may campaign for a seat on a district hospital board or be asked to serve by a religious leader. Certain people start with duty as a primary reason and later move from a sense of obligation to a state of real enjoyment in their role as board members.

Representation. This is a reward when the hospital's bylaws state that certain geographic areas are allowed a seat on the board. Some church hospitals have representatives from each congregation, for example, a historical remnant of the days when each church provided financial support to keep the hospital solvent.

Appointment. In some cases the mayor, the town council, or the governor appoints people to serve. This method results in certain board members who are there for someone else's reason rather than their own, but some political appointees I've known have far exceeded expectations. When they are chosen, this conveys a "select status" that in political circles is very meaningful.

Power or influence. If all board members wanted were satisfaction and a chance to give service, they could volunteer in
many less conspicuous ways. But there is a real "electricity"
near the seat of power. The closer the better, and the board
members get to make major dollars-and-cents decisions.
What's more, good board members don't shy away from ac-
knowledging this. It is a major reward for many of the good
people who serve.

The legacy effect. Many board members want to leave
something of themselves behind. Few board members can en-
dow a building or major physical facility that would bear their
name after they die, but collectively working with fellow directors they can leave their mark, whether on a brass plaque or
in the corporate minutes.

Satisfactions of Service

Different individuals on the same board will be guided by
vastly different motivations. For example, two attorneys may
sit on the same board. One is entirely motivated to serve for the
recognition she'll get in the media, as she is contemplating
running for political office. The second attorney, a man with
inherited wealth, might practice law to keep busy and serves on
the board because of influence, prestige, or to make a contribution to community affairs.

The point is, board service offers real satisfaction and
rewards for an individual. If the board on which an individual
serves is organized, focused, and well-directed, the benefits
multiply. When boards select members for their specific talents, skills, and interests and then add the training and direction necessary, they've created a highly favorable environment
for individual growth.

Every board can improve its operation and performance. I
hope that tangible methods have been presented in this book to
stimulate board and management thinking to explore the
board's role.

The dynamics of the group and the world in which health care is operating will change constantly. It's easy for board members to mistakenly think that one board is just like any other board. My personal and professional experience has shown exactly the opposite. Boards are unique and hospital and health care boards are also different from other types.

Simple things are, at times, very difficult. Whether it's golf, tennis, bowling, or making a soufflé, professionals make it look easy. But they practice the basics every day. For those who only occasionally try to perform the job, it can be difficult and complex.

An Action Agenda

Board members can help to build a better board if they are willing to:

— Accept the fact that trained management will lead and the board will oversee by various methods.

— Constantly clarify the mission of the organization and realize their job is to keep that mission alive for board members, management, medical staff, and the public.

— Define in detail the job and responsibilities of the board. This will allow better definition of what type of persons are needed for the future.

— Re-explore board mechanics to help break routines and rituals, keeping the board from becoming bored.

— Evaluate the board's performance. This is only possible when the board is mentally mature enough to be self-critical.

— Better define the board chairperson's role, to make this into a more meaningful and less ceremonial position.

— Hire, evaluate, and motivate the CEO. These are the board's greatest responsibilities.

— Make sure the medical staff practices medicine and management practices management, with the board serving as overseer.

In Conclusion

The voluntary hospital organization has been the most successful not-for-profit enterprise created in our society. It has brought together concerned citizens, highly trained professionals, and management to achieve remarkable results. Medical technologies alone have spawned thousands of for-profit businesses and specialized professional services. While the system has been effective, it has also produced excesses and abuses. Government and other payers are today creating the kinds of pressures that will again reshape hospitals.

The board of directors is theoretically charged with seeing that wise decisions are made in the community's best interests. As the rules of the game are changing in favor of competition rather than voluntary cooperation, new director perspectives will be needed. Some boards will be threatened by the change and will try to ignore realities, while others will be revitalized and thrive.

Will your board be capable of changing how it operates? Or will efforts to strengthen the board's organization and procedures be stifled? Will new standards of performance be threatening to the long-term volunteer? Will pay for performance on boards of directors create a holier-than-thou attitude or will it bring new skills to the boardroom? Will physicians be salaried employees in your health care organization in the future or will yours be the last organization with private practice physicians?

To keep up with management and medicine, boards will need to move boldly in new directions. The shift to better, stronger boards of directors has already begun and it will gain momentum in this age when health care is increasingly judged more by its financial performance than by its compassion.

When a majority of hospital boards decide to clarify their

roles and purposes and to enforce new standards of performance, this industry will experience immense change. I feel the
greatest untapped potential in hospital organizations is in the
board. Hospital management today has "closed the gap" between health care and general business. Medical science continues to explore exotic, life-enhancing technologies. Only
boards still function a generation behind the times.

Change is not easy. But the rewards for structuring a new
board of directors to face the new health care world will be
satisfying and fulfilling beyond anything boards have yet experienced. *You* can build a better hospital board, and I wish you
well in the effort.

Appendix A

Mission Statements

Evangelical Health Systems
Oak Brook, Illinois

Mission

The mission of Evangelical Health Systems (EHS) is to provide for the effective and efficient delivery of quality health care and health-related services in areas of identifiable need, for the benefit of individuals, families, and society. In keeping with its heritage and philosophy, EHS is committed to maintaining a Christian emphasis in all its endeavors.

Goals

To carry out the healing ministry of Jesus Christ, the EHS emphasis on Christian ideals will be of primary importance in guiding the operations of the system.

— EHS expresses its Christian philosophy throughout its range of activities.

— EHS affirms its United Church of Christ heritage and will support a continuing relationship with all constituencies of the church to fulfill its mission in meeting the health care needs of society.

— EHS health care services are provided regardless of religious belief.

— EHS will continue to provide health care to the economically disadvantaged and will act to improve access to health care and improve the quality of life for all individuals, commensurate with its resources.

— EHS will provide leadership in the area of medical ethics.

EHS will strategically coordinate the resources of all subsidiaries to effectively provide a broad range of health care and health-related services.

— EHS will foster the wellness of individuals through a comprehensive range of health care services that respond to a person's physical, emotional, and spiritual needs.

— Policies and procedures, consistent with the organization's philosophy, will be established to ensure that all services offered by the system are of quality, are cost-effective, and are technologically current.

— An integrated strategic plan will be implemented to maximize the effective allocation of resources. Specifically, this market-based plan should enable EHS to provide leadership in the health care industry and meet human needs.

EHS will manage its financial affairs to meet goals and objectives while maintaining the flexibility to adapt to external changes that may affect the organization.

— EHS will maximize utilization of its resources by seeking to efficiently allocate them to fulfill its mission, achieve productivity gains, and minimize health care costs.

— EHS will ensure the continued financial viability of the system through the establishment of financial guidelines. These will require: (1) an adequate return in order to finance growth and diversification while maintaining and replenishing the capital resources of the organization; and (2) a prudent level of business risk through diversification, debt management, and the establishment of adequate reserves.

EHS will seek to maximize the availability and quality of its human resources (including governance, volunteers, medical staff, and employees) through effective recruiting, development, and retention of such personnel without regard to race, religion, sex, or age. To achieve this goal, EHS will:

— Provide a holistic work environment conducive to individual effectiveness, positive morale, effective two-way communications, and opportunities to career development.

— Emphasize educational and development programs for all human resources, including governance, the medical staff, volunteers, and employees.

— Implement equal opportunity programs to promote the recruitment and advancement of minorities.

— Promote from within EHS whenever possible.

— Recruit qualified personnel from outside EHS when necessary.

— Institute procedures to ensure continuity of management.

— Provide an equitable and competitive level of compensation for employees.

In keeping with its philosophy, EHS will assume specific community-related responsibilities.

— EHS and its subsidiaries will keep abreast of community health care needs and, where feasible, implement plans to help meet these needs.

— The parent company and its subsidiaries will engage in appropriate clinical and administrative research activities consistent with patient care requirements and available resources.

— EHS will fulfill its responsibilities of corporate citizenship—both within the communities served by its institutions and within the system's greater service area. EHS will, where appropriate, encourage its employees and medical staff to assume positions of leadership in such organizations as trade associations, planning bodies, and various citizens' groups.

— EHS will monitor federal, state, and local legislation to keep abreast of issues that could affect health care and the organization. In this process it will seek to establish its governance, management, and medical staff as knowledgeable resource personnel who can assist in helping formulate legislation and regulatory rules that are in the best interests of the health care field and society.

Relationship Statement between the Central Texas Annual Conference and the Harris Methodist Health System Fort Worth, Texas

1. Introduction. The Harris Methodist Health System is a coordinated multi-institutional health care and related services system in the north-central area of the state of Texas. The System was originally created as an expression of the health and welfare ministry of the Central Texas Annual Conference of the United Methodist Church, and it continues to share the beliefs, goals, and purposes of the Conference and the Christian church. Its work is the physical expression of the Christian church's underlying human compassion for those in need. The health care facilities and services provided by the institutions within the System are available directly or by referral on an inpatient and ambulatory basis for the medical needs of persons in the area they serve. It is the belief of the System that institutions of healing are an essential aspect of the ministry of the Christian church, having its origin when a Galilean carpenter brought healing to the blind, the lame, and the helpless. It is His Spirit that has been behind every effort to heal the sick, and it is still His compassion and love that brings health to the whole person. There is no healing of the human body that is complete without the healing of the human spirit, and it is this spiritual dimension that sets the Christian hospital apart from others. Medical technology, which has come through divine guidance and is administered through a Christian health care institution which makes its services available to all in need, is mankind's hope for a healthier tomorrow.

2. The service area. The area served by the System is the geographic territory extending approximately 150 miles to the north, west, and south of Fort Worth, Texas. Specifically, the System's prime service area is composed of the following counties: Archer, Baylor, Bell, Bosque, Brown, Callahan, Clay, Coleman, Comanche, Cooke, Coryell, Dallas, Denton, Eastland, Ellis, Erath, Freestone, Hamilton, Hill, Hood, Jack, Johnson, Lampassas, Limestone, McLennan, Mills, Montague, Navarro, Palo Pinto, Parker, Runnels, Shackleford, Somervell, Stephens, Tarrant, Throckmorton, Wichita, Wilbarger, Williamson, Young, and Wise.

3. Relationships within the System. The System consists of an affiliated group of non-profit and for-profit health care and health care support organizations, all of which are controlled, directly or indirectly, by Harris Methodist Health System, a Texas non-profit corporation, which is the parent organization. The System looks to the Central Texas Annual Conference of the United Methodist Church as a source of spiritual guidance and as a source of interested and qualified persons who will support the missional goals and respect the high standard of care and operation of the System. The members of the board of directors of the System are elected by the Central Texas Annual Conference, and 25 of the 32 members are required to be active members of the United Methodist Church. However, the board of directors of the System is not amenable to the Central Texas Annual Conference. The board of directors has exclusive authority over and responsibility for all corporate activities of the System. The Central Texas Annual Conference has no authority over or responsibility for any financial or legal obligation of the System. Neither shall the System have any authority over or responsibility for any financial or legal obligation of the Central Texas Annual Conference.

4. The member health care institutions. The following health care institutions are presently included within the System: (1) Harris Hospital-Methodist, a special care and general acute care hospital in downtown Fort Worth, Texas; (2) Harris Hospital-Hurst-Euless-Bedford, a special care and general acute care hospital in Bedford and Euless, Texas; (3) Harris Hospital-Eagle Mountain Area Suburban Hospital, a general acute care hospital in Azle, Texas; (4) Dublin Medical Center, a general acute care hospital in Dublin, Texas; (5) Decatur Community Hospital, a general acute care hospital in Decatur, Texas; (6) General Mexia Memorial Hospital, a general acute care hospital in Mexia, Texas; (7) Stephenville General Hospital, a general acute care hospital in Stephenville, Texas; (8) Meridian Hospital, a general acute care hospital in Meridian,

Texas; (9) Meridian Geriatric Center, a nursing home located in Meridian, Texas; (10) Marks-English Hospital, a general acute care hospital in Glen Rose, Texas; (11) Glen Rose Nursing Home, a nursing home located in Glen Rose, Texas; (12) Hamilton General Hospital, a general acute care hospital in Hamilton, Texas; and (13) Memorial Hospital-Cleburne, an acute care hospital in Cleburne, Texas.

It is recognized by the System that from time to time hospital affiliations may be changed or altered. The above list is not intended to represent a limitation. Rather, it is anticipated that new health care facilities will be added to the System as its health care ministry expands.

Each proposed affiliated institution will be within or in immediate proximity to the service area; will have the clear capability to become financially viable on its own merits; will assure the System that there is a broad-based community consensus of the desirability for affiliation; will have the potential to provide a high quality of patient care equal to that of the other affiliated hospitals in the System; and will provide for a means to dissolve the affiliation should it be necessary. It is the System's steadfast goal to produce net revenues available for debt service equal to at least 110 percent of the System's total principal and interest requirement for each fiscal year.

5. The health care mission. The System will provide high quality health care to its patients in a manner as economical and efficient as possible without regard to race, religion, or sexual status, and without regard to financial status subject to the indigent care budget of the System. This includes maintaining and, when appropriate, improving, modifying, or creating medical, ancillary, and diversified support services; expanding shared services arrangements; affiliating with other institutions through management contracts, lease agreements, or purchase; developing health services delivery programs; and implementing preventive and restorative programs through health education and promotion. The System will maintain high competency among medical, nursing, clergy, management, and allied health personnel. Clinical education opportunities for medical, nursing, clergy, and allied health personnel will be provided by the System through its affiliated institutions. Medical education programs at each affiliated institution will be approved by each institution's medical staff. Research projects will conform to the policies and procedures of each affiliated institution.

In support of this health care mission, the Central Texas Conference shall, in turn, provide moral and financial assistance to the System's charity care program (Golden Cross) through a Golden Cross offering taken annually among all of its member churches.

Miami Valley Hospital
Dayton, Ohio

Miami Valley Hospital, as a component of MedAmerica Health Systems Corporation, supports the fulfillment of MedAmerica's mission by providing quality, cost-effective health services for citizens of the Greater Miami Valley Region.

While carrying out this mission, Miami Valley Hospital shall enhance its role as the region's preeminent health care service provider by delivering individualized patient care and service for the total person through:

— Innovative, effective programs designed to meet the health care needs and wants of the consumer.

— A comprehensive range of services, including selected tertiary services uniquely available at Miami Valley Hospital.

— Staff of competent, caring physicians and employees who respect personal dignity.

— Comfortable and convenient facilities, with modern medical equipment.

— Competitive prices offering high value for the services purchased.

— A commitment to its religious heritage.

— Selected professional and community health education programs that enhance health care in the region.

— Assured access to appropriate health services for all persons with a life-threatening or incapacitating condition, regardless of ability to pay.

— A productive work environment that promotes excellence and seeks to maximize the quality of work life of all physicians and employees, without discrimination.

Appendix B

Board Job Descriptions

St. Catherine Hospital
Garden City, Kansas
The Role of the Board of Directors

A few years ago people felt very honored and eager to be appointed or elected to the board of directors of a hospital. However, the drastic change in the role of the board now causes people to think seriously before accepting the job. What is the reason for their hesitancy?

While it is true trusteeship means guardianship or stewardship and a hospital is a service/social institution serving the people of God in a community, a hospital in 1984 is a business confronted with governmental regulations. It exists in a competitive environment with other hospitals and an increasing variety of alternative health care delivery agencies and organizations. To survive in such an environment, a hospital must engage in risk ventures.

Consequently, the role and qualifications of a board member have shifted. A new level of commitment and business expertise in trusteeship is needed if the established values of hospital care are to be meaningful, quality care monitored, and lawsuits avoided.

Some of the functions of St. Catherine Hospital Board of Directors are the following:

— To ensure that the sponsoring group's philosophy is implemented.
— To establish broad hospital policies and provide for a continual review of such policies.
— To approve the selection of a qualified medical staff.
— To evaluate all phases of hospital performance, including the quality of medical care.
— To approve financial and other major reports prepared by hospital personnel.
— To ensure that the community's health care needs are met.

Although the board has the responsibility for the hospital's performance, it does not operate the hospital. The day-to-day operation is the function of the hospital administration. The administrators manage the hospital and report on its operation to the board of directors.

Therefore, it is imperative that hospital board members be people who can perceive the role of governance clearly, avoid conflicts of interest, conceptualize policy questions, be aware of health services from a community standpoint, understand professionalism, encourage forward-looking strategies, and have a genuine interest in the health needs of the community. Only then will the hospital have a viable future.

St. Joseph Health System
Orange, California
December 1984
Job Description for Affiliated Board Trustee

Position: Board Trustee of Affiliated Corporation
Reports to: Chairperson of the Affiliated Board
Directs: CEO of the Affiliated Corporation

Summary of Responsibility

Collectively, the board of the affiliated corporation is responsible for the implementation of the mission and philosophy, and the management of the business, property, and affairs of the affiliated corporation, subject to the reserved rights of its corporate member. More specifically, the board is responsible for the direction of the corporation, and its continued viability in the health care ministry; establishment of plans, policies, and programs for the corporation; provision of guidance to the affiliated CEO; the quality of health care delivered in the organization; preservation and replenishment of assets; rendering all decisions not reserved to the corporate member; compliance with statutory requirements; and the transfer, through the System CEO to the corporate member, of issues falling under rights reserved to the corporate member.

If the affiliated corporation is the corporate member of one or more subsidiary corporations, then the board of the corporation will be responsible for ensuring that the subsidiary corporation(s) adheres to all applicable System policies. The board of the affiliated corporation will also be responsible for developing, implementing, and monitoring the working relationship with the subsidiary corporation(s).

Individually, each trustee of the affiliated corporation is responsible for participation in the accomplishment of board responsibilities and the maintenance of positive internal and external relationships and an image consistent with the mission and philosophy of the Sisters of St. Joseph of Orange. Each trustee serves the interest of the Congregation, the System, and the affiliated corporation as a whole, rather than serving only a particular area or function.

Responsibilities

Participates in the approval and submission of long-range plans to the corporate member that will ensure implementation of the mission and the viability and continuity of the affiliated corporation.

a. Maintains an understanding of the mission and philosophy of the Sisters of St. Joseph of Orange and their applicability to current health issues and the affiliated corporation.

b. Maintains current knowledge of major developments in:
   — Environmental factors as they affect health care.
   — Health delivery trends and structures.
   — Health financing trends.
   — Multihospital corporations.
   — Catholic-sponsored institutions.
   — Health care legislation.

c. Provides input to the planning process about such matters as community needs, the reputation and standing of the corporation, activities of competitors, threats to the mission and philosophy, and opportunities for enhancing the institution's goals.

d. Ensures that affiliated corporation long-range plans reflect and are consistent with the mission and philosophy of the Sisters of St. Joseph of Orange and the strategic plan for the System.

e. Approves long-range plan(s) for recommendation to the corporate member.

f. Ensures that criteria and standards are established that will allow evaluation of plan implementation.

g. Reviews annually the long-range plan and confirms its direction or proposes a change of direction to the corporate member.

Participates in the development of services and resources needed to implement long-range plan(s) and achieve the purpose of the affiliated corporation.

Organization and Authority

1. Ensures that the organizational structure of the corporation facilitates the implementation of its plan and realization of its purpose.

2. Reviews and approves major changes in relationships (authority/accountability) with the corporation.

3. Ensures that program and service delivery structures are appropriate to meet community needs given corporate resources.

4. Establishes those controls deemed necessary to protect properly the rights and interests of the Congregation, employees, medical staff, patients, and creditors.

5. Approves the bylaws of the medical staff organization.

6. Approves the granting of privileges for physicians to practice at the institution.

7. Monitors the quality of care provided by the corporation. Ensures that medical care meets accepted standards.

8. Approves the revocation of privileges or other corrective action against members of the medical staff.

9. Authorizes officers to sign various written instruments and to take financial action.

10. Appoints individuals who can act for the affiliated corporation.

11. Approves the establishment/abolishment of board committees.

12. Periodically evaluates the performance of board committees.

13. Annually reviews bylaws and recommends changes to the corporate member.

14. Approves the annual reports.

15. Performs all duties imposed by statutory requirements or the bylaws.

Fiscal

1. Ensures the prudent preservation and timely replenishment of corporation assets.

2. Approves annual operating budget and capital budget that are consistent with and supportive of the long-range plan of the corporation and the mission and philosophy of the Congregation. Recommends the budgets to the corporate member for approval.

3. Recommends to the corporate member the purchase, sale, lease, disposition, or hypothecation of real property by the affiliated and subsidiary corporations.

4. Approves short-term financing up to 20 percent of the average monthly total operating revenues for the preceding fiscal year or $500,000, whichever is greater. Recommends larger amounts to the corporate member for approval.

5. Recommends to the corporate member the approval of any long-term financing for the affiliated and subsidiary corporations.

6. Approves contracts and purchase agreements not otherwise approved in the budget process for the

affiliated and subsidiary corporations up to $100,000. Recommends larger agreements to the corporate member for approval.

7. Approves the acceptance of donations whose conditions do not significantly affect the nature, purpose, plans, or identity of the affiliated corporation and that do not necessitate capital expenditures in excess of $50,000. Recommends all other contributions to the corporate member for approval.

8. Approves the establishment of reserves for the corporation.

9. Approves investments for the corporation.

10. Approves charitable contributions to the church, charities, etc.

11. Receives and reviews annually a report on insurance coverage.

12. Examines the financial reports on a periodic basis to identify and obtain explanations for:
   — Variances from budget.
   — Significant trends.
   — Impact of objectives and goals on financial position.
   — Impact of financial performance on objectives and goals.

Human Resources

1. Participates in the CEO selection process as outlined in the selection procedure. Recommends to the corporate member the discharge of the CEO.

2. Recommends to the corporate member the removal of board trustees for sufficient cause.

3. Provides input to the System CEO in the process of CEO evaluation.

4. Ensures development of personnel in the corporation, including those sisters who serve there.

5. Ensures that new board trustees and other key personnel are oriented to the Sisters of St. Joseph of Orange, the System, and the affiliated corporation.

6. Ensures that trustees, officers, and other corporation employees act in accordance with established ethical and professional standards.

7. Seeks improvement in own management and leadership skills.

Facilities

1. Recommends to the corporate member the approval of the purchase, sale, lease, disposition, or hypothecation of real property.

2. Ensures that facility and site provisions are adequate to allow implementation of long-range plan(s).

Consultation

1. Receives reports of pending legal or ethical charges against the corporation that are likely to result in substantial loss of reputation or money.

2. Receives reports of all substantial ongoing or potential litigation brought on behalf of the corporation.

3. Through the CEO, notifies the System office of all charges or litigation referred to above.

4. Through the CEO, consults with the System office on all charges or litigation referred to above.

Participation in Board Activities

a. Attends board meetings of the affiliated corporation.

b. Formulates corporation plans, policies, and standards

in board committees regarding mission, philosophy, human resources, fiscal performance, quality of care and work life, and response to community needs.

— Attends committee meetings and chairs committees as appointed by the chairperson of the board.

— Works with board committee members and staff to the committee.

— Ensures that agendas are developed, meetings scheduled, and minutes recorded and disseminated for those committees that are chaired.

— Ensures that policies are consistent with and supportive of:

1. The mission and philosophy of the Sisters of St. Joseph of Orange.
2. The strategic plan of the System.
3. Policies.
4. Corporation plans and policies.

— Presents policy recommendations to the board for approval.

c. Reviews, modifies, and votes on plan, policy, and program proposals.

d. If elected, serves as an officer of the board.

e. If chairperson of the board, serves on the executive committee.

f. Advises and gives counsel to the CEO.

g. Reviews corporation performance against purpose, plans, policies, and objectives.

h. Inquires into performance deficiencies and takes corrective action as required.

i. Reviews minutes of meetings to identify follow-up action required, research to be completed prior to the next meeting, and issues not fully resolved.

j. Processes reserve rights issues for the corporate member.

k. Reviews and comments on System plan, policy, and program proposals.

The Efficient and Effective Operation of the Board

a. Contributes to the maintenance and development of a helpful, caring, and professional climate within the board.

b. Contributes to a climate of openness and service to others.

c. Maintains confidentiality of board and System activities as appropriate.

d. Exercises fiscal constraint in the fulfillment of board duties.

e. Performs other tasks as assigned by the chairperson of the board.

Establishment and Maintenance of Effective Relationships

a. Maintains an effective relationship with the Congregation of the Sisters of St. Joseph of Orange.

— Contributes to the development of the statement of mission of the System and subsequent goals, plans, and policies.

— Integrates the mission and philosophy into the direction, policies, programs, and services of the corporation.

— Forwards issues falling under rights reserved to the corporate member through the System CEO.

- — Ensures that requests from the Congregation are honored courteously and promptly.
- — Ensures the prevention of social and fiscal jeopardy to the Congregation and the affiliated corporation.

b. Maintains positive relations with the medical staff.

c. Ensures that positive relations are maintained between members of the medical staff and staff of the institution.

d. Assists in establishing and maintaining positive external relations with:

- — Government agencies.
- — Church agencies.
- — Other health care providers.
- — Civic and community organizations and associates.
- — Appropriate businesses and industries.

Index

About the Author

JOHN A. WITT is a well-known consultant and speaker throughout the health care industry. During the past 25 years he has delivered hundreds of speeches and seminars to health care executives and board members. As proof of his acceptance, he has been invited back to many organizations time and time again.

Mr. Witt simultaneously educates, entertains, and stimulates his audiences with practical suggestions for change. Whether as a keynote speaker or as a seminar leader, he challenges his audience to think and to grow.

His consulting firm pioneered ethical executive search and training programs for boards of directors in the health care industry. His ideas, predictions, and thoughts occasionally raise eyebrows, but a look back frequently proves the wisdom of his words.

Mr. Witt started his career with Allis Chalmers Manufacturing Company; he soon moved to St. Luke's Hospital in Milwaukee, Wisconsin. After several years there, he traveled nationally for the American Hospital Association and later for A.T. Kearney, as a consultant. In 1969 he formed a search firm specializing in health care, which became the largest specialty search firm in the entire country.

He has written and spoken on all phases of health care management. His columns have appeared in two national health care monthlies read by thousands of executives and board members.

Mr. Witt received his Bachelor of Arts degree from Luther College, Decorah, Iowa. He is a member of the American Association of Healthcare Consultants, the Association of Executive Search Consultants, and the National Speakers Association.

Thus begins John A. Witt's classic commentary, *Building a Better Hospital Board*. Witt, the consummate consultant, has drawn upon his 25 years of work in health care organizations to write a book with meaning and significance for board members and senior management in health care alike.

Witt begins with a discussion of leadership, pointing out the different roles of the board and the chief executive and how governance is the appropriate board posture. Next he examines the hospital's mission statement, the cornerstone of the board's whole program. He suggests methods for directors to remain zealous in pursuit of the mission. Samples of actual mission statements are appended.

Following is a review of an "elite" board that includes 10 guides to selecting the best board members and some thoughts from Witt on the housekeeping details of board organization. He suggests that hospital boards meet quarterly — for two days — instead of several hours per month. And, he suggests that board members be paid for their service — a controversial concept.

The responsibilities of a board member and some sample job descriptions are covered next, followed by an examination of the issues related to board performance evaluation. Several sample formats for evaluation are provided. Next is a discussion of the board chairperson's role. Witt feels this area has been too long neglected, as the chairperson can make or break an organization.

All of Witt's years as an executive search consultant are brought to bear on chapters that detail the process of hiring, evaluating and compensating the chief executive officer. He calls hiring the CEO "the board's single most important task," and ranks evaluation and compensation issues right behind. Employment contracts and benefits packages are reviewed from the board's viewpoint, and he offers counsel on keeping the CEO motivated through a variety of techniques.

The board's relationship with the medical staff is reviewed in a chapter that focuses on the historic role of the physician in the hospital and looks to the future as new relationships emerge.

Finally, Witt applauds those who serve on hospital boards, and provides food for thought as he lists the motivations for this

'07